Karen S. Geiser and Lisa J. Amstutz
foreword by David Kline

Local Choices

Join the local foods movement! Easy practical steps to:
A healthier you.
A greener planet.
A stronger community.

D1113014

ISBN 978-1-933753-16-4

Book Design | Brenda Troyer
Printing | Carlisle Printing of Walnut Creek

Carlisle Press
WALNUT CREEK

2673 Township Road 421
Sugarcreek, Ohio 44681
phone | 800.852.4482

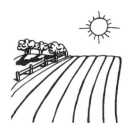

Acknowledgements

We are grateful for the technical support and encouragement of our husbands, the patience of our children (who love their veggies with the dirt still hanging on), the many friends who shared their stories, and to God, whose creation we are stewarding.

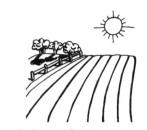

Table of Contents

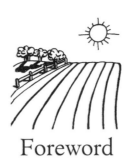

Foreword

All my life as a farmer and "helper in the garden," most of the food on our table traveled less than half a mile from its roots to our table. In fact, I still find it hard to find an empty tin can for worms when I want to take the grandchildren fishing. Almost everything we eat, if not fresh, was canned, cured and smoked, dried, or frozen here on the farm. In a sense, the minerals in the bones and bodies of our family come from the soil of our 120 acres.

Growing our own food was and is easy because we have the land and good soil that nurtures plants, animals, and humans. For many people it isn't so simple and it could be for a number of reasons—poor soil or lack of space for a garden, time, or possibly even the knowledge of gardening and the preparation and preservation of "unprocessed foods."

In this book, *Local Choices*, authors Lisa Amstutz and Karen Geiser gently address this difficulty. Instead of plunging into local and home-grown foods at full throttle, a more small-scale approach is offered. Convert a corner of a small flowerbed into a two- or three-plant tomato garden, which requires very little effort. Buy a little cold frame and grow lettuce for salads. Blend your own dressings for the salads. Experiment. Surprise your spouse and family with your exotic creations. As you gain confidence in your abilities as a gardener and chef, expand your garden. Watch your thumb. As it turns greener, enlarge your plot.

The choice to go local and your decision to buy this book is likely multi-faceted. It is in all probability a combination of economics, health-consciousness and wellness, getting your hands into the tilth of fertile soil, putting a face on your food, and good taste.

What can compare with a garden-ripened tomato, zaftig with juice, on a summer's evening?

On the other hand, if you are intimidated by the thought of planting your own garden, you should perhaps think about buying a share in a local CSA (Community Supported Agriculture). Community Supported Agriculture (in Canada it is called Community Shared Agriculture) is well explained by the authors in this book.

My wife Elsie had a small CSA of six to ten families during the 1990s. Every Thursday afternoon was pickup day here at the farm. She would place, freshly harvested, what was available that week on an octagon picnic table in the shade of the sweet cherry tree and the members would make their own choices on what they needed.

Most of the afternoon was spent visiting around that table while their children would explore the farm or go swimming in the pond. Usually the items on the table included some non-vegetables such as fresh eggs, new honey, oven-fresh bread, and toward fall, apples from the orchard. This also provided an excellent opportunity to learn not just about our different cultures but also about gardening: the best flavored and disease-resistant varieties, when to plant the fall garden (the first ten days of August), heirloom vs. modern tomatoes for canning, preparing the best sweet corn (steam the ears set on end, don't boil them), and what gourmet food really is.

What Elsie's CSA members soon realized, somewhat to their surprise, was how weather-connected farmers are since we were a non-irrigating farm. If the rains were timely and gentle, the gardens flourished and the picnic table abounded with weekly vegetables. If it didn't rain for several weeks, the varieties and abundance dwindled and the members began to understand the capriciousness of farming.

If even the thought of how to adequately use hundreds of dollars' worth of vegetables from a CSA overwhelms you, consider visiting the local farmers' market, talk to the producers and ask questions, and then buy only small amounts of produce—vegetables that don't need a lot of preparation, such as radishes and carrots. Fresh radishes, lightly salted, on buttered wheat bread is kings' fare.

I believe most of us would agree that quality of life begins at the table. But then, food is more than just nourishment for the body, it is also the time when family and friends and even strangers gather around the table to share in the goodness of the fields and gardens.

Amstutz and Geiser bring together the necessity and goodness of eating locally in this well-thought-out and nicely done book. They use the knowledge and wisdom of many people, from Henry Thoreau to their neighbors.

I invite the readers of this book to engage their family, friends, neighbors, and community to follow the authors' example in eating locally and eating well. As Karen writes about their 78-acre farm, "Our livelihood is dependent on having customers committed to making us their regular grocery stop. In some ways, writing this book is a plea to keep small farmers like ourselves in business by educating others on the benefits of making the effort to find foods locally."

- David Kline
Author, Farmer, Naturalist

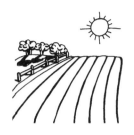

Introduction

An Invitation to the Local Table

There will come a day when a carrot, freshly observed, will spark a revolution.
-Paul Cezanne

This book was conceived over a cup of local mint tea shared by two small-scale farmers one quiet winter day. We found that we shared a growing desire to help more people discover the joys and benefits of eating local food, as we both have done at our family tables. There are some excellent local foods books on the market, but we felt one was missing: an easy-to-read volume that could help even the busiest person to take just one step toward eating closer to home. *Local Choices* gives an overview of the local foods scene, offers tidbits of research, shares personal experiences from farmers, and most importantly, relates abundant stories from real people who are including local foods in their diets.

We believe that the "eat local" trend is more than just a fad—it is a movement that is here to stay and may someday be a matter of survival in a world with fluctuating oil and food prices. This movement has sometimes been criticized as an elitist trend, where the well off feast on swanky gourmet food and luxury items that common folk can't afford. *Local Choices* refutes this misconception by bringing together stories of ordinary people who believe in the value of eating local and are making it a priority for their family. Most of our contributors are of average income (some well below average). They come from many walks of life and represent a variety of food philosophies, from strict vegetarian to committed carnivore. They have made sacrifices to choose foods that affect their health, their communities, and their world in a positive way.

WHAT DO WE MEAN BY EATING LOCALLY?

In the United States, the average food travels over 1500 miles before it reaches our dinner plates, and the typical prepared meal boasts ingredients from five countries. U.S. farms have been disappearing at a rate of 219 per day for the past 50 years.[1]

However, a small but growing group of concerned consumers are bucking these trends. This group is often referred to as "locavores," or "localvores"—people seeking to eat food grown close to home. For some, the concept of "eating local" means religiously searching out foods grown within a 100-mile radius of their home. There are websites, local chapters, and books dedicated to this concept. For others, "local" means simply purchasing food from their own state or surrounding states rather than food shipped across the country or from abroad.

Here in northeast Ohio, we could go to the supermarket and purchase white bread, peanut butter, jelly, potato chips, and ice cream—all of which are arguably "local." Several large, well-known food corporations produce those foods near our homes. But is eating this way really eating local? We don't think so. While each of these companies does a good job of hiring local workers and treating them decently, they are still sourcing their ingredients from hundreds or thousands of miles away and processing them almost beyond recognition. For the purposes of this book, we will define eating local as eating foods that are locally grown and produced, in season, and minimally processed. When possible, we recommend organically or sustainably grown fruits, vegetables, and grains, and pastured meats and dairy products. We believe this way of eating is better for the earth, better for our own health, and better for the health of our local economies.

WHY WOULD ANYONE WANT TO EAT LOCAL?

We surveyed over 50 people who intentionally source some of their food locally. We asked them what motivated them to make these

---

1 Leopold Center for Sustainable Agriculture, "Checking the Food Odometer," July 2003, *New Scientist*, Oct. 9, 2004.

changes, and found that there were a number of common factors. Health is a big motivator, including both the fear of contamination and a desire for more nutritious food. Some were sold on eating local when they realized that fresh food tastes better. Others were moved to action when they became aware of the overall effect their food choices have on the world and on future generations, or when their religious beliefs inspired them to make changes.

As we talk with friends and customers, we sense that many are longing for authenticity and genuine connections with their food, but don't know how to find it in this world of 24-hour superstores, strip malls, and all-you-can-eat buffets. Most of us have lost the food cultures that originally sustained us, with the exception of a few special holiday treats, passed down as family traditions. Barbara Kingsolver writes, in *Animal, Vegetable, Miracle*, "At its heart, a genuine food culture is an affinity between people and the land that feeds them. Step one, probably, is to live on the land that feeds them, or at least on the same continent, ideally the same region. Step two is to be able to countenance the ideas of 'food' and 'dirt' in the same sentence, and three is to start poking into one's supply chain to learn where things are coming from."[II] As we begin to discover the foods growing all around us, we forge a connection with and appreciation for the places where we live and the people who grow those foods for us.

NAVIGATING THIS BOOK

The first two chapters of this book give an overview of some of the reasons people are choosing local foods and the advantages of local foods to you and your community. In chapter three, we move on to practical ways to put these concepts into practice. Each chapter includes a list of steps to take and recommended resources if you'd like to dig deeper on individual topics.

There's an old riddle that goes, "How do you eat an elephant?" The answer, of course, is, "One bite at a time." There is a kernel of truth in this joke—a seemingly impossible undertaking becomes quite

---

II Kingsolver, Barbara, Camille Kingsolver, and Steven L. Hopp, *Animal, Vegetable, Miracle: A Year of Food Life*. (HarperCollins: 2007) 20.

possible when broken down into bite-sized chunks. And so it is with the steps we recommend in this book.

Our hope is that you will take one step—one forkful—one minute to consider. And that one meal at a time, you will begin to create a more joyful food culture for yourself and your family and friends. We're not looking to make you feel guilty or deprive you of your favorite foods, but rather to introduce you to a new way of eating that will make your mealtimes increasingly meaningful, healthful, and earth-friendly. Make *Local Choices*!

- Karen S. Geiser

- Lisa J. Amstutz

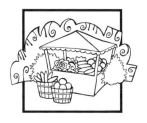

CHAPTER 1

The Benefits of Local Foods

Tell me what you eat, and I will tell you what you are.
- French gastronomist Anthelme Brillat-Savarin

A MATTER OF TASTE

Last winter, Lisa's family received a most unusual e-mail from one of our egg customers. Our free-ranging, backyard flock lays fewer eggs in the winter months, inspiring this humorous attempt to egg them on: "Dear Hens... My mornings are colorless since I can no longer open a box of eggs with brown, blue, and green tinted shells. My son's chocolate chip cookies are less creamy without your rich yolks. My world's no longer sunny-side up, but scrambled and sad—please start laying!"

Now I am almost certain that the average hen has never received any fan mail. She labors anonymously in her small cage, churning out perfect, uniform eggs without even a "thank-you." So what is it about these eggs that inspires such devotion? Well, they are certainly beautiful, with their variously colored and speckled shells, but when you get right down to it, what really makes these eggs e-mail-worthy is their flavor. Farm-fresh eggs from pastured hens have a depth of flavor that most North Americans under the age of fifty have never experienced.

Flavor is one of the primary reasons that people choose local foods. Over the past fifty years or so, many of us have grown accustomed to less-flavorful foods, and have come to rely heavily on added sweeteners, salt, and flavorings to compensate. In the name of convenience, we've settled for TV dinners, casseroles-in-a-box, mushy canned peas, and iceberg lettuce with about as much flavor as its namesake. We are so used to this fare that many of us don't even realize what's missing. We have forgotten, or never learned, what a fresh, juice-dripping homegrown tomato tastes like, or a freshly laid egg, or a sticky-sweet, perfectly ripe peach. We have forgotten how good real food can taste.

The Slow Food movement emphasizes "the right to taste." This movement has over 80,000 members worldwide. According to www.slowfood.com, "By reawakening and training their senses, Slow Food helps people rediscover the joys of eating and understand the importance of caring where their food comes from, who makes it, and how it's made."

Our friend Lori had a peach epiphany that awoke her interest in local foods:

> For years my family struggled to eat the firm, tasteless peaches sold at our local supermarket. Since they were rock-hard when we brought them home, we tried to ripen them (as directed) in a paper bag on the counter. Despite our efforts, the peaches never ripened but rotted instead. Frustrated, we stopped buying peaches until the day I happened upon a local peach orchard. My family and I devoured these peaches—sweet, velvety, and fragrant—with juice running down to our elbows and collars. Each of us ate several peaches a day, hungering after the delicate flavor and texture only a "picked-ripe-off-the-tree" peach can offer.
>
> The taste, smell, and texture compelled us to savor the joy of the moment, but it also soothed something within our souls. This was real food! We realized that eating could be a richer experience if we chose to abstain from the firm, tasteless food offerings at the local supermarket and went searching for ripe, recently picked food. It was an epiphany moment that inspired us to search for local food.
>
> When neighbor children are over during peach season, of course peaches from our local orchard are offered for a snack. Most refuse, saying they don't like peaches. Our children will beg them to try just a bite, assuring them it is not like any other peach they have tried. The neighbors are usually pleasantly surprised to find that they like peaches after all.

FRESH PEACH SALAD

6 ripe peaches   1 C. fresh blueberries
1 C. vanilla yogurt   pinch of cinnamon and nutmeg

Slice peaches and mix with blueberries. Blend yogurt and spices. Stir into fruit or use spiced yogurt as fruit dip. This is a great mid-summer treat when both peaches and blueberries are in season.

–Lori S.J. is a schoolteacher and mother of two. She also runs a small soapmaking business from her home in the suburbs. Lori and her family eat mostly vegetarian meals, sourced locally when possible, and see their food choices as a practical expression of their faith and values.

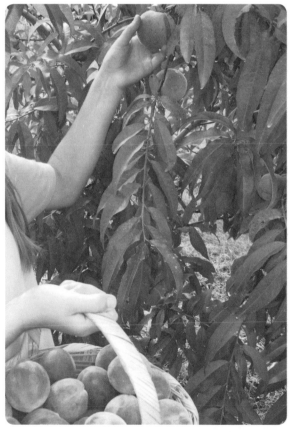

Nothing beats the flavor of tree-ripened fruit. When you buy from a local orchard, chances are your fruit was picked that day and will be bursting with flavor.

TOO MUCH TRAVEL TIME

Part of the reason our modern foods lack flavor is that we are growing them increasingly farther from home. The food on the average North American dinner plate has traveled at least 1500 miles, a fact which does not bode well for its flavor. Most supermarket fruits and vegetables are picked green because we need them to survive their long journey, several days in the grocery store, and a few more in our refrigerators. Sometimes the packaging contains chemicals to delay ripening. Upon arrival, exposure to ethylene gas in large ripening rooms causes the ripening process to resume.[1] Many items are still not fully ripe when we buy them at the supermarket—bananas are often green, and peaches, pears, and avocados are hard as rock. Unfortunately, although they will eventually soften and change color, most fruits and vegetables will never fully develop their flavors when they ripen off the plant.

Even in fully ripened produce, flavor and nutrient content decline after harvest. Sugars quickly change to starches after harvest, and vitamins and other compounds gradually break down. This is why freshly picked corn on the cob tastes so much better than ears shipped across the country, and why fresh backyard asparagus beats the supermarket version hands down. The shorter the time from the field to the table, the more sugars and flavors remain.

Freshness affects the flavor of eggs, milk, and meat as well. Like fruits and vegetables, these foods lose quality with every passing day. Many people find the superior taste of fresh, local foods to be well worth the extra effort required to track them down.

INDUSTRIAL-STRENGTH VARIETIES

In addition to its untimely harvest and long road trip, globetrotting food has to survive rough handling. That out-of-season supermarket tomato was likely mechanically harvested, tossed on a conveyor belt and bounced around on a refrigerated truck before reaching your plate. It takes a strong constitution to survive this ordeal, so fruits and vegetables are increasingly bred for durability and uniformity rather than lip-smacking flavor.

---

1   "Stop Putting that Produce in the Fridge!" from Fresh Food Central, http://www.freshfoodcentral.com/view_feature.aspx?featureid=6.

Such a breeding scheme would have been inconceivable to our great-grandparents, who carefully selected seeds from their most flavorful fruits and vegetables, swapped with neighbors, and saved for the next year. They developed an astounding number of varieties. Baker Creek's 2008 heirloom seed catalog lists 165 kinds of tomatoes, 24 kinds of radishes, and 37 types of cucumbers, for example. In recent years, small growers have snatched many of these varieties back from the brink of extinction as agribusinesses focus more and more on a few industrial-strength varieties.

This year we grew two varieties of Patty Pan squash: Green Tint (light green) and Sunburst (yellow). Chefs like them when they are about the size of a half dollar, but they can be used at any size. They have a mushroom-like flavor and are stuffed with cheese and baked. You can also dip the flowers in egg, roll in flour, and fry them. One customer liked them at a more mature stage because she liked the seeds. Patty Pans are rarely found at grocery stores, especially with their flowers still attached. At the farmers' market this year, we had requests for just the blossoms themselves. (See fried bloom recipe below and Patty Pan squash recipe in Appendix A.)

We planted our Ambrosia yellow raspberries last spring. They produced enough this year for us to sell at the market. Most people have never seen yellow raspberries and are unaware of any varieties other than red and black. These berries are less acidic than red raspberries and have an apricot taste. We found that whether the fruit is large or small, our berries have a lot more flavor than store-bought varieties.

FRIED PATTY PAN BLOOMS

Pick open or closed blooms from your squash plants. Gently rinse and roll in a paper towel to dry. In mixing bowl, beat two eggs. In separate bowl, measure ½ C. flour. Melt equal parts butter and olive oil together in a sauté pan and heat. Dip the bloom in the egg and then roll in the flour. Place blooms in sauté pan and fry for several minutes. Once they are browned, remove and place on a paper towel on a plate.

–Sisters Rachel and Deb G. own Pioneer Farm in Kidron, OH. They use sustainable farming methods on their small-scale farm and sell their products at a local farmers' market and an on-farm store. Rachel and Deb enjoy growing unusual heirloom varieties of fruits and vegetables. They also raise laying hens, bees, and heritage turkeys.

While heirloom varieties are fun (and even addictive), you don't need to eat unfamiliar things to enjoy the flavors of fresh foods. Many small farmers also raise traditional modern varieties, such as Blue Lake beans, Big Boy tomatoes, and red potatoes. When grown nearby and harvested at peak ripeness, these old favorites still wield a flavor advantage over their out-of-state competitors.

Eating locally may sound like self-denial—after all, your options will be limited and you may have to wait all year for your favorite foods to come into season again. However, by choosing to eat seasonally you can experience a new depth of flavor and discover a different kind of variety.

PAY THE FARMER OR PAY THE DOCTOR

Health issues are a perennial hot topic in the media, and we are beginning to realize the role that food plays in keeping us healthy. We increasingly witness this trend at the Geiser farm as many of our produce customers' health concerns drive them to seek out local, unprocessed foods. One season we served several pregnant mothers concerned with nourishing their growing little ones, a recovering cancer patient who is very careful to avoid chemicals, a long-time customer with a diabetic husband, and someone with rheumatoid arthritis who uses fresh herbs and produce from our farm to reduce her need for pharmaceuticals. Several customers are concerned about the nutritional value and chemicals in their children's food, while others are working at weight loss.

Bev S., a high-school teacher, realized after the serious illnesses of several family members that she needed to be intentional about healthy eating and living. She has committed herself to buying less processed foods and recently tried eggs and pastured poultry from our farm. According to Bev, the chicken tasted like "real chicken;" she hopes she never has to eat flavorless store eggs again; and she is eager to learn what other farm products we have available. Her inability to fit all the foods she wants into her limited budget also inspired her to start tearing out landscaping plants in order to try growing produce on her small lot in town. Overall, Bev has been pleasantly surprised to find that adding local, healthful foods to her diet has not been a deprivation, but rather a tasty and fulfilling process. Another local food aficionado commented, "I consider myself a frugal and wise consumer. When it comes to food, I'll cut corners in other areas so I can buy good food because I believe good food isn't cheap and cheap food isn't good. High-quality food really is cheap medicine and I'd rather visit the local farm stand than the pharmacy any day."

To be sure, local food isn't automatically healthful, but it is likely to be less processed, with fewer harmful additives. At the farmers' market, it is easier to find locally grown potatoes than potato chips, and freshly ground flour than Twinkies. Author Michael Pollan offers simple advice on choosing healthy foods. He urges people to cook and eat fresh foods, find local produce, and avoid unpronounceable ingredients and processed convenience foods. Don't buy things "your grandmother wouldn't recognize as food," he says, like portable tubes of yogurt with fifteen ingredients. Don't eat anything that won't rot. And don't buy foods that make health claims, which are usually boxed, processed, and supported by big marketing budgets.[2]

Honey, maple syrup, sorghum molasses and fresh stevia are all natural sweeteners you may find at local markets. Replacing white sugar with these natural options takes some adjustment but can have a positive impact on your health. In most cases, you can substitute honey, molasses and maple syrup at a half cup per cup of sugar in any recipe. You may need to increase the amount of dry ingredients to achieve proper consistency. Fresh or dried stevia is a good way to sweeten tea and other beverages. If you are uncomfortable figuring out substitutions, we recommend *Healthy Choices* Cookbook (Carlisle Press, 800.852.4482) which contains recipes without white sugar, white flour or artificial ingredients.

NUTRIENT DENSITY

Even fresh produce may be lacking in nutrients, as long commutes from the field to the table result in vitamin loss and protein breakdown. This gives an advantage to food that is grown nearby and hasn't spent days in transit before reaching your kitchen. Changes in farming practices have also caused declines in nutrition. In today's world, broccoli is not broccoli is not broccoli. A growing body of research

---

2 Kenning, Chris, "Author Cites 'National Eating Disorder,'" *The Courier Journal*, January 12, 2008.

shows that the food value of plants directly relates to soil nutrient level, cultivar choices, and other factors. Donald Davis, a biochemist at the University of Texas, has documented declines in the nutrient values of fruits, vegetables, and wheat of 6-38% over the last 50 years. Other studies show nutrient decreases of up to 60% in meat and dairy products.[3]

Breeding for efficiency results in jumbo, fast-growing fruits and veggies. However, such fast-ripening foods may not be able to uptake nutrients as fast as their smaller-sized relatives due to their shorter lifespan and smaller root mass. Conventional farming practices also lessen the nutrient concentration of foods. Nutrients must be present in the soil in order for the plant to uptake them. A fundamental concept of ecological farming is "Healthy soil equals healthy food equals healthy people."

As we grew older, we became a lot more health-conscious. When someone close to you gets cancer or has heart disease or diabetes, you begin to think about causes, and food and diet become an important consideration. One of my relatives is a naturopath and advocates eating organic foods—which can be an expensive proposition if you don't have a local source. As someone who grew up on a small family farm, I started to realize how my habits of shopping and eating have contributed to the demise of many farms and how our food industry has influenced health. For instance, most processed and packaged foods turn out to be poor substitutes, health-wise, for the original—compare corn chips with fresh corn on the cob, or supermarket tomato sauce with homemade marinara from your garden produce.

I've become an advocate for eating *natural* foods and so I am more likely to use a reasonable portion of butter rather than some processed grocery item. I mix it with olive oil and try to use some of the skim and low-fat cheeses rather than a steady diet of high-fat products. We eat many vegetarian meals, which taste amazingly good when you make them with fresh, local produce. I think my husband and I are healthier

3   Donald R. Davis, PhD, FACN, Melvin D. Epp, PhD, and Hugh D. Riordan, MD, "Changes in USDA Food Composition Data for 43 Garden Crops, 1950 to 1999." *Journal of the American College of Nutrition*, Vol. 23, No. 6 (2004) p. 669-682.

than many of our contemporaries who aren't as "into eating well" as we are. One problem is that our food tastes so good, we eat more than we should!

–Joanne L. is an author, writing teacher, and grandmother who enjoys writing about her garden as much as eating from it. She shares garden space and chores with an Amish neighbor.

ASK THE FARMER

You might not be able to identify by sight an "empty" cabbage from a nutrient-rich one, but if it has been grown locally, you have the opportunity to ask the farmer more about how it was grown and make an informed decision about your purchase. On the Geiser farm, one of our goals is to make our food as nutritionally dense as possible. We add compost, shredded leaves, and calcium to our one-acre market garden. We grow cover crops to protect the soil from erosion and add nutrients, and apply concentrated seawater that contains a full complement of elements. In addition, we rotate crops each season and leave some areas to rest for a year with only a cover crop.

Our philosophy in raising animals is to give them access to the food and lifestyle that they are suited for to ensure that their products are as nutritious as possible. Our Hereford beef cattle eat the

> *CLA, or conjugated linoleic acid, is most abundant in meat and dairy products from grass-fed animals. The level of CLA in these products is three to five times higher than comparable products from grain-fed animals. CLA shows great promise in the battle against cancer. ~www.eatwild.com/healthbenefits.htm*

grass and hay that their ruminant stomachs are designed to digest. The cattle move to a fresh paddock of pasture daily during the growing season and receive a supplement of mineral-rich kelp.

Research on the content of omega-3 fatty acids and CLAs in grass-fed meat products versus their grain-fed counterparts confirms the value of our methods (see sidebar). Our laying hens take dust baths and roam the pasture to supplement their diet of grain mash with clover, grasses, and bugs to yield eggs with deep orange yolks and whites that have distinct edges. The broilers move about on pasture and yield meat that many describe as tasting the way chicken used to taste when they were young. Our family Jersey cow lives on lush grass and provides our family with creamy milk for butter, yogurt, cheese, and other vitamin-packed dairy products.

Our jump into full-time farming has proved to be a very satisfying way of life but has not been without its bumps and challenges. We are thankful to live on our 78-acre family farm and to be able to work together outdoors as a family doing things we love.

Small-scale farming does involve risks—weather damage to a crucial crop, livestock tragedies like losing chickens to predators, and even the necessity of a part-time winter job to keep the bills paid are all part of the reality of farming.

Much of our work in the market garden and pastures is done by hand or with older equipment, so we cannot compete with the efficiencies of a mega-farm with thousands of acres and all the latest technologies. We are still learning what crops and animals are profitable for our time and situation. Because of the thought and effort put into production, we trust that the food we produce is of highest quality and will lead to good health for our customers. However, comparing our hourly wages with those of healthcare professionals is sometimes discouraging.

Our livelihood is dependent on having customers committed to making us their regular grocery stop. In some ways, writing this book is a plea to keep small farmers like ourselves in business by educating others on the benefits of making the effort to find foods locally.

OVERWEIGHT AND UNDERNOURISHED

Have you ever noticed that the more unhealthy foods you consume, the more you crave? Bruce Ames and other researchers are studying a condition they term "hidden hunger," which results from a diet that is deficient in micronutrients. In developing nations, diets consisting of only a single kind of grain may cause this hidden hunger. In industrialized nations, it often results from a diet of cheap, processed foods. Ames says that people who eat these types of diets are "starving for vitamins and minerals." Although they may eat enough (or even too many) calories, their nutritional needs are not being met. [4]

---

4   Messinger, Leah. "Cellular Nutrition : The Hunt to Fix Hidden Hunger," SFGate. com, December 17, 2006. http://articles.sfgate.com/2006-12-17/living/17326513_1_ pesticides-ames-test-carcinogens.

Gail's story would seem to back up this hypothesis and was one of my (Karen's) most satisfying experiences as a farmer. Gail is a single mom in her upper forties who was facing serious health conditions and struggling to pay her bills, which included expensive medications. She contacted local agencies for help but found that food pantries simply did not offer the fresh fruits and vegetables that the doctor had recommended to help her lose weight. Through a church secretary who is one of our regular produce customers, I connected with Gail and began taking weekly baskets of extra produce to her. As our friendship grew and she made progress in losing pounds, I was motivated to add more good food to her weekly baskets, like pastured eggs and meats as well as a fresh bouquet to feed her soul.

> *Omega-3's are 2-4 times more abundant in meat from grass-fed animals than meat from grain-fed animals. Studies show they aid in the prevention of heart attacks, cancer, Alzheimer's, depression and more. (www.eatwild.com/healthbenefits.htm.)*

Over the course of seven months, with admirable self-discipline, Gail was able to lose over 70 pounds. We both agree that having easy access to good, nutrient-dense food played a large role in her success. She also claims that the flowers were as valuable in that process as the food. One of my long-term visions is to help establish a food pantry filled with healthy staples and fresh vegetables in season so that more people like Gail can thrive.

"Let your food be your medicine and your medicine be your food" is the famous mantra of Hippocrates, the father of modern medicine. We believe that Hippocrates' philosophy still holds true today. Our hope is that someday farmers' markets will be busier places than doctors' offices, headlines about obesity will be obsolete, and the farmer growing nutrient-dense foods will receive the same respect in society as the physician caring for the ill.

IS YOUR FOOD SUPPLY REALLY SAFE?

Food safety is not a fun topic, but it's an important consideration for consumers who want to make informed decisions about their food. Our food is being raised increasingly far from our homes—in many cases, beyond our borders—and we have no reliable way of knowing how it is grown. We eat grapes from Chile, kiwis from New Zealand, and garlic from China. In this industrialized, dehumanized system, we have no choice but to put our faith in labels and the ability of our government to protect us from unscrupulous or unsanitary producers and processors. Unless, of course, we can find a trusted supplier and meet them face to face.

We spoke with a county health commissioner who concurs. "One result of the industrialization of our food supply is concentration of processing plants and the increased potential of contamination from poor oversight, accidents, or intentional acts," said Dr. D.J. McFadden. "The best way to solve this, in my opinion, is to move toward a system of more small family farms where there is a relationship between farmer and consumer. If this doesn't happen, increased careful government oversight is definitely a necessity for consumer safety."

BACTERIAL CONTAMINATION

Seventy-six million Americans are sickened every year by food-borne illnesses. Five thousand of them die.[5] In 2007, the USDA recalled more than fifty products due to contamination, and the FDA recalled many more. Some of these recalls were massive enough to put entire companies out of business. Many others, however, barely made the news.

E. coli O157:H7 is a common culprit in outbreaks of food-borne illnesses. While some E. coli occurs naturally in the gut of humans and animals, this particular strain can cause deadly illnesses and long-term health problems.[6] The increase in this strain has been linked to the way cattle are raised—specifically, the practice of feeding them grain when their ruminant digestive systems were designed to consume grass. Very little E. coli O157:H7 is found in grass-fed cattle, but feeding them grain, ethanol by-products, and other foods that nature did not intend for cattle to live on makes for a more acidic gut—just the conditions that E. coli O157:H7 prefers.[7]

---

5   "Hot Topics: Health & Food Safety", www.foodroutes.org/hottopic.jsp?id=2.

6   Centers for Disease Control and Prevention listing, http://www.cdc.gov/nczved/divisions/dfbmd/diseases/ecoli_o157h7/

7   Diez-Gonzales, Francisco, Todd R. Callaway, Menas G. Kizoulis, James B. Russell. "Grain Feeding and the Dissemination of Acid-Resistant Escherichia coli from Cattle". *Science*, Vol. 281. No. 5383, September 1998: pp. 1666 – 1668.

E. *coli* problems are not limited to beef products. Infected cattle can contaminate produce if their manure comes into contact with crops or irrigation water. Bacteria can even be taken up into the plant itself, where they cannot be washed off. Because processing of greens is so centralized—as Michael Pollan aptly put it, "we're washing the whole nation's salad in one big sink,"—any bacteria that slip in can taint the whole batch and sicken people nationwide.

> When the *E. coli* spinach scare came along, we were thankful that our supply of spinach was in our backyard. When we hear about Mad Cow disease and other meat safety issues we are glad to know that our beef and chicken is coming from healthy animals at a local farm, though we are still looking for a reliable source of pork.
>
> I think in both cases (the spinach and beef), my realization of the advantage of a local, known source of food came while watching the news. The news stories seemed to project fear and concern and I was struck by a sense of peace of mind and security. And thankfulness. When it comes to raising young children, the world offers enough fear and concern as it is, without having to worry about what they are eating. The "extra" cost of planting and picking the spinach was well worth it. If the beef cost a little more also, what is the price of peace of mind?
>
> *–Mark B., a technician at a wood products shop, is the father of two preschoolers who relaxes by working in his backyard garden. Mark's family especially enjoys using fruits from local orchards and each year they try something new to add to their repertoire of produce that they preserve for winter eating.*

Many other bacteria can cause illness, including *Listeria, Staphylococcus aureus, Camphylobacter,* and *Salmonella*. Overcrowding, stressful conditions, and lax sanitation favor the growth of these bacteria. We asked Mike Mariola, chef and owner of the South Market Bistro in Wooster, Ohio, for his thoughts on food safety. "When I think about food safety, I think about a lot of the issues in the past couple of years in the media, and all of them stem from not knowing the food system that you're getting products from," he said. "I just find a lot of comfort in buying locally. I don't have any concern about dealing with any of our farmers. I've been out to all their farms.

I know where they package their product, I know how they store it and transport it, and I'm comfortable with all of those. They will look me in the eye when they drop a product off and I know that they are dropping off a great product."

PESTICIDE DANGERS

As the mother of several apple-loving children, I (Lisa) was horrified to learn that 8% of conventional apples contain so much pesticide residue that half an apple exceeds FDA safe exposure levels for a two-year-old.[8] According to the EPA, children are more vulnerable than adults to the effects of pesticides (chemicals applied to wipe out insects, weeds, or fungi from a field) due to their smaller body size and still-developing bodies.[9] Eating pesticide-laden food increases pesticide levels in the body. The good news is that eating organically grown foods quickly reduces those levels.[10]

Here again it is important to note that *local does not equal organic*. When it comes to pesticides, the chief advantage of buying locally grown food is the ability to ask the growers about their pesticide usage and make a fully informed decision.

Not-so-sweet strawberries: *"Strawberries get doused with 350 lb. per acre of toxins, including some that are among the most dangerous to farm workers, the environment, and consumers."*
- *Kimbrell*

Many of the safety issues mentioned above stem from the efficiencies and large scale of industrial agriculture. Though locally produced foods are not immune to food safety problems, any outbreak caused by them would at least be small and localized. All these threats of contamination are scary, but as an informed consumer, you can make safer choices.

8   Kimbrell, Andrew. *Fatal Harvest* (Foundation for Deep Ecology: 2002) 164.

9   United States General Accounting Office Report to Congressional Requesters, PESTICIDES: Improvements Needed to Ensure the Safety of Farmworkers and Their Children. March 2000. www.gao.gov/archive/2000/rc00040.pdf.

10   Lu, Chensheng, Kathryn Toepel, Rene Irish, Richard A. Fenske, Dana B. Barr, and Roberto Bravo. "Organic Diets Significantly Lower Children's Dietary Exposure to Organophosphorus Pesticides," *Environmental Health Perspectives*, Volume 114, Number 2, February 2006. www.ehponline.org/members/2005/8418/8418.html

GENETICALLY MODIFIED FOODS

Unless you eat 100% organic or homegrown foods, you probably eat GMOs (genetically modified organisms) every day. You are part of one of the largest experiments ever conducted on unknowing participants. An Ohio State University fact sheet states that 60-70% of food products in the United States contain genetically modified ingredients, the most common of which are corn and soy.[11] The FDA does not require labeling for genetically modified foods, unlike the European Union, Japan, China, New Zealand, and many other countries.

GMOs are created in specialized laboratories where scientists take specific genes from one organism and insert them into another in hopes of producing a certain trait. The two combined organisms may be completely different from each other—plants can even be implanted with bacterial or animal genes. Many times companies select for traits like herbicide resistance so that herbicides can be applied without killing crop plants, but scientists have also attempted to make foods healthier as well. The oft-cited "golden rice" is an example, where researchers created a strain of rice with higher levels of vitamin A in hopes of curing deficiencies in developing countries. In another, markedly unappetizing experiment, roundworm genes were transferred into pig fetal cells to create a "heart-healthy" pig with increased levels of healthy omega-3 fatty acids.[12] Of course, a much simpler way to achieve this would be simply to graze the pigs on pasture; grass-fed animals in general have much higher levels of omega-3s than their grain-fed counterparts.

Food allergies are a concern in relation to genetically modified foods. If genes from an allergenic food are *A four-digit PLU number means that produce is conventionally grown (not organic). Organic produce has a five-digit number beginning with nine. A five-digit number beginning with eight means the item is genetically modified (GM).* inserted into other foods, the resulting proteins could cause an allergic reaction—and no warning label is required on genetically modified

---

11   Sereana H. Dresbach et al., "The Impact of Genetically Modified Organisms on Human Health," http://Ohioline.osu.edu/hyg-fact/5000/5058.html.

12   Gina Kolata, "Cloned Pigs Could Provide Meat That Benefits the Heart," *New York Times*, March 26, 2006. www.nytimes.com/2006/03/26/health/26cnd-pig.html?_r=2&ei=5070&en=1.

foods unless the FDA is aware of such a link.[13] In addition, the new forms of proteins created by genetic engineering could potentially create new allergies.

Eyewitnesses note that animals often avoid GM foods when given the choice. Studies on animals have documented health problems such as bleeding stomachs, liver and pancreas problems, and inflammatory effects resulting from GM feed.[14] Some of these studies still need to be replicated; however, they give cause for concern and should call for more in-depth research before GM foods are released.

GM foods generate complex issues that go beyond the grocery shelf. Spreading pollen can contaminate nearby crops, heavy herbicide usage on GM crops is creating "superweeds," and the possibility of a few large corporations controlling the world's seed supply is an alarming prospect. It is a complex topic that warrants further study by concerned consumers (see resource list).

BIOTERRORISM AND NATURAL DISASTERS

The more globalized our food system becomes, the more vulnerable we are to bioterrorism. Our country's agriculture is now so centralized that nearly all of the processing takes place in a few giant plants, and the vast majority of the vegetables produced in the United States come from a small number of mega-farms. This means that every one of these farms carries the potential for thousands of people nationwide to be sickened if contaminants were to be intentionally introduced into the system.

In addition, globalization leaves us vulnerable to supply chain failures in the event of an electrical outage, natural disaster like Hurricane Katrina, or oil shortage. In many areas, there is simply no food available if the supply chain fails. Imagine what would happen in your area if no out-of-state trucks could get through. What would you eat? We can work to increase our food security by growing and buying food in our own regions. A pantry full of preserved foods and a backyard garden can provide food security for your own family and

---

13   Dresbach et al., "The Impact of Genetically Modified Organisms..."

14   The Health Risks of GM Foods: Summary/Debate, -http:/www.seedsofdeception. com/Public/GeneticRoulette/HealthRisksofGMFoodsSummaryDebate/index.cfm.

others in times of emergency and a network of nearby family farmers can help secure our food supply even in a crisis.

The primary benefit for our family from eating locally is health. Knowing the source of my food, what chemicals were or were not used in production, and the increased nutritional content are important to us. It's also nice not having to peel certain fruits or vegetables to avoid the chemicals. Then we get the added nutritional content of the peeling.

A more recent motivator is the thought of what I would do in the event of an economic/military/transportation/weather disaster, and how I could ensure that my family eats healthfully during such a crisis. In addition to keeping a good supply of our own preserved vegetables, I have been establishing where I can get various foods—especially staples like flour, rolled oats, honey, dairy, and eggs (ensuring that it is actually produced locally and not dependent on a supplier)—even if my budget cannot presently support getting it there.

–Jolene M. is the mother of three preschoolers. She makes it a priority to seek out local, organic foods. As her children grow older, she hopes to expand their small backyard garden to keep their food supply close to home. Until then, she continues to read and learn from other gardeners.

LOSS OF VARIETIES

Loss of diversity is leaving us extraordinarily vulnerable to crop failures. Historically, genetic variety has protected humanity from starvation—when disease, insects, or weather wiped out one crop, another one took its place. Much of the breeding that we have done in the past century has relied heavily on variation in both wild and cultivated varieties. Heavy reliance on a single variety has very real dangers, as the Irish discovered in 1845. Many families at that time depended on potatoes, and specifically on one variety, the lumper, for their survival. When a new fungus (the potato blight) arrived from North America, the entire potato crop was wiped out and hundreds of thousands starved.[15] Millions more left the country.

---

15   Japikse, Catharina. "The Irish Potato Famine of the 1840s," *EPA Journal*, Fall 1994. www.victoryseeds.com/news/irish_famine.html

As any gardener can attest, nature abhors a monoculture. Yet monoculture is exactly what industrial agriculture encourages. Most of the plant-based foods we eat (over 75%) derive from just nine crops. Many of the fruit and vegetable varieties that existed in 1900 are now extinct. For example, 80-92% of all tomato, lettuce, field

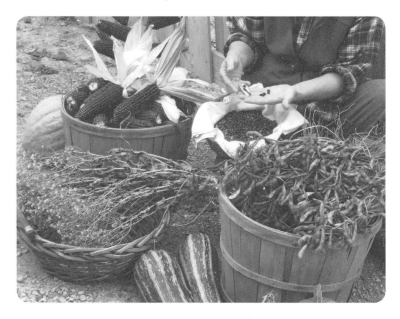

Farmer Amy S. continues the ancient tradition of seed saving. By perpetuating her own Bloody Butcher corn, Fortex beans, and Italian zucchini, she saves money and preserves genetic diversity in her market garden.

corn and apple varieties have disappeared.[16]

There are seed banks and other groups working to prevent further loss of varieties, but the best way to "save" varieties is to purchase, plant, and eat them, thereby making them profitable for nurseries to grow. The opportunity to save these varieties lies with individual gardeners/farmers and consumers who want diverse products.

We never run out of wonder in our seed-saving experiments. I couldn't resist ordering the 18 varieties of heirloom tomatoes I'm growing for the CSA garden this year. If variety

16   Kimbrell, 71.

is the spice of life, then the garden is my nirvana. Orange carrots, green bell peppers, and white cauliflower are just too boring for our family now that we've grown red carrots, orange peppers, and purple cauliflower. I say, "Bring on the purple potato French fries, and don't spare the green zebra catsup!"

This year I will have Brandywine seed that has adapted to our soil for over seven years...they just keep getting better. This has been so hope-giving that I just cannot resist adding new varieties each year. I figure, if I can inspire one more person each year to save another tomato variety, my grandchildren might be able to enjoy a persimmon, or a garden peach in their tomato patch someday.... now that's living!

–Amy S. and her family own the Simon Certified Organic Family Farm in East Sparta, OH, where they offer a CSA, herd shares, and grass-fed meats. They love to experiment with heirloom varieties and educate their customers on how to use them. Winter finds them drooling over seed catalogs and attending farming conferences as they plan for the next season.

STEPS TO TAKE

1. Research health issues and their relationship to food. Substitute a fresh, local product for a processed food in your diet. Some good places to start: replace sugar with local honey, boxed snack foods with local apples or homegrown carrots, or soda pop with local tea.

2. Visit the FDA website and check out the list of recent recalls. Investigate local sources for some of the most frequently contaminated foods in recent news—beef, spinach, and lettuce.

3. Go beyond vegetables and look for local sources of meat, milk, and eggs, noting labels like free-range, grass-fed, hormone-free, etc. Purchase a small amount for your family to sample.

4. Play detective and research the growing conditions of a local food product you purchased: ask the farmer, surf the web, etc. to learn about farming practices, soil health, and more.

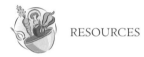

RESOURCES

1. *Real Food: What to Eat and Why* by Nina Planck

2. *In Defense of Food: an Eater's Manifesto* by Michael Pollan

3. *How to Pick a Peach: The Search for Flavor from Farm to Table* by Russ Parsons

4. *Fatal Harvest* by Andrew Kimbrell (Editor)

5. *Holy Cows & Hog Heaven* by Joel Salatin

6. *Pasture Perfect* by Jo Robinson or www.eatwild.com (information on grass-fed meat and dairy products)

7. *Food, Inc.* DVD by Robert Kenner

8. The Weston A. Price Foundation (whole foods in the traditional diets of many cultures)

9. *Healthy Choices Cookbook* by Marvin and Miriam Wengerd, Carlisle Press. 1800.852.4482

COOKING WITH HERBS

Culinary herbs add flavor to your food, and many contain unique nutritional properties. Due to their fragile nature, herbs quickly lose quality and flavor so they are best purchased fresh at the farmers' market or picked right in your backyard. Most can even be grown indoors on a sunny windowsill. Here are some basic herbs to get you started:

Basil - This spicy herb is the epitome of summer flavor. It can be chopped fresh and sprinkled on tomatoes, salads, or pasta dishes. Make a simple pesto by whirling 2 cups of basil leaves, ½ cup olive oil, 2 cloves garlic, ½ cup Parmesan cheese, and ¼ cup pine nuts or walnuts in the blender. We often make a big batch when basil is in season, freeze it in ice cube trays, and then transfer the cubes to a plastic freezer bag. This makes it easy to pull out a cube as needed for winter meals.

In general, herbs will keep for a few days with their stems in a glass of water in the refrigerator, or wrapped in a damp paper towel inside a plastic bag in the crisper drawer. Basil leaves, however, can turn black in the fridge, so a countertop bouquet is best for short-term storage.

Parsley - Italian flat leaf or curly parsley both give a mild, fresh green flavor to food and combine well with other herbs. Soups, meats, and veggies are enriched by adding a handful of parsley. Raw, chopped parsley can also be sprinkled on salads and other dishes for a distinctive tang.

Chives - The long slender stems of chives may be chopped and sprinkled on baked potatoes, rice dishes, and omelets for a delicate onion flavor. Toss a few of the purple blossoms on salads to add flavor and color.

Rosemary - The distinct piney flavor of rosemary goes well with many meats. Sprinkle whole stems over a roasted chicken or lamb roast. Chopped rosemary is delicious tossed with olive oil on potato wedges and baked at 400° for 45 minutes.

Dill - Use the feathery greens, flower heads, and seeds to season salads, dips, creamy sauces, and breads. Dill pickles and potato salad spiked with dill are other tasty options.

Mint - The many members of the mint family give a fresh lift to cold fruits, ice cream, and salads. Steep a handful of fresh or dried leaves in hot water for a refreshing hot or iced tea.

CHAPTER 2

Voting with Your Fork

How we eat determines to a considerable extent how the world is used.
- Wendell Berry

Deeply held values motivate many people to choose local and sustainably grown foods. These values include care for the environment, the safety and treatment of agricultural workers, and the health of local communities. For some, religious values are part of the equation. In this chapter, you will find stories of people who have chosen to shop and eat in a way that lines up with their values and are, in effect, voting with their forks for the kind of world they want to live in.

We are motivated by a desire to live more richly and do our part to take care of our bodies, our communities, and the earth. Knowing where our food is coming from, what hands and methods are used to grow it, keeping our money in our local economy and straight into the hands of the farmer and not a bunch of intermediaries, tasting an egg laid by a hen that is loved like a pet—these are ways of living we value.

I see my choices as my vote of how I would like the world to be. Although my choices may not seem to make a difference in the grand scheme of things, it is one thing I can do to make a difference. I believe in supporting local people. I believe in choosing foods grown in ways that take care of our earth and aim to preserve it for future generations. If money talks, then I will use it to buy items that contribute to the stewardship of our bodies and the earth. Everything has a cost—it just is not always money. I try to look at the long-term costs/effects of all my choices.

~*Lori S.J.*

ENVIRONMENTAL IMPACT

Consider a typical breakfast of toast with butter and jam, coffee, and orange juice. Before reaching my table, the orange juice has traveled from Florida and the coffee from Central or South America. My favorite supermarket bread comes from another state, so it has logged double miles as the ingredients traveled first to the factory and then in packaged form to my grocery store. Since I live near a jam factory, the jam may not have traveled far in its processed form, but its ingredients have already traveled thousands of miles to reach the factory.

On the other hand, I could prepare almost the same meal with vastly fewer food miles. I could make bread with flour from a nearby farm, or buy bread from the neighborhood bakery, topping it with homemade or farmers' market jam made from local ingredients or local honey. I could replace the orange juice with grape or apple juice, both of which grow here in Ohio. Tea from a local tea farm could replace the coffee or I might treat myself to some Fair Trade coffee.

While dining on ethnic cuisine can be an enjoyable treat, basing our everyday meals on such distant sources is clearly unsustainable. A tremendous amount of fuel is required to transport each of those foods from their sources to our homes. Here in Ohio, we can grow apples, peaches, nectarines, and strawberries, along with many other fruits and vegetables. Yet supermarkets persist in importing these fruits from California, Washington, Michigan, etc.—even while they are in season here. Meanwhile many of our Ohio-grown foods are feeding people in other states or countries. This whole system is incredibly fuel-inefficient. By contrast, you can buy an apple or strawberry at a farmers' market or roadside stand that has traveled only a few miles at most. Author Steven Hopp points out that eating one local, organic meal per week per person would save our country over 1.1 million barrels of oil a week.[17]

> Every choice we make in farming is based on our values. Our goal is to build the human and natural communities. We work at that by providing fresh, healthy food for people and producing it in a way that increases, not degrades, environmental health. Some may look at what we do and think it takes too much hand labor, that we could do it easier or in greater volume with more machinery or with chemicals. But that makes no sense to us. We're trying to reduce our impact on the planet—produce fewer harmful emissions, release fewer poisons—and farming with organic techniques is the best way to do that.

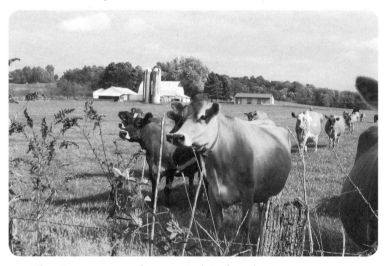

These Jerseys are part of an organic dairy farm that incorporates grazing as part of their feed program. Grass-based farming reduces fossil fuel usage, improves animal health and results in healthier foods.

> Selling our produce locally is a way to serve our local community. Not only does it provide good food to our neighbors but it also builds great relationships. Some of

---

17   Kingsolver, Barbara, Camille Kingsolver, and Steven L. Hopp, *Animal, Vegetable, Miracle: A Year of Food Life.* (HarperCollins: 2007) 5.

our best friends now are members of our CSA (Community Supported Agriculture) and farmers' market customers. Growing and selling local food builds community.

~Ron & Mary M. own and operate Strawberry Hill Farm in Fresno, OH. The farm supplies 35 CSA customers and a weekly farmers' market with seasonal produce and eggs. Mary works from home part-time as an editor for a small publishing house.

Industrial foods require oil for more than just transportation. On large-scale farms, petroleum is involved in every aspect of tilling, planting, spraying, and harvesting. From there, vast amounts of oil are consumed in food processing (milling, sorting, baking, drying), packaging (plastics are made from petroleum), and energy used for storage and cooling. According to some estimates, our current system of agriculture uses seven to ten calories of energy to produce one calorie of food energy.[18]

> "*It takes 36 calories of fossil-fuel energy to grow and ship 1 calorie of iceberg lettuce. 'We might as well be shipping baggies of water back and forth across America,' says Bill McKibben."*
> -Bob Schildgen,
> "10 Ways to Eat Well," Sierra, Nov/Dec 2006

Fae M., a retired nurse and mission worker, is enthusiastic about how little packaging she uses when she buys local food. "Besides the benefit of more tasty and nutritious food, I appreciate that I can purchase items with less packaging," she writes. "Many of the baskets and cartons can be reused several times and the organic wastes can be turned into compost. I believe in recycling everything I can with very little trash for the garbage man to pick up, and buying foods locally helps me accomplish that."

CARING FOR THE SOIL

Most of us don't give much thought to soil; at least not in positive terms. The words we associate with it—soiled, dirt, dirty, dust, etc.— have negative connotations; they sound unhealthy and undesirable. Perhaps we need a new vocabulary that recognizes the beauty and importance of this miraculous substance. Descriptive words like loam, sand, silt, and humus help us look more carefully at our soil and

---

18   "Fossil Fuel and Energy Use," www.sustainabletable.org/issues/energy.

describe it more accurately. Changing how we look at and think about the soil can help us learn to care for it and treat it with reverence.

Properly caring for the soil reduces the need for synthetic fertilizers and pesticides and reduces the amount of oil needed to produce our food. Stewardship of the soil also ensures the continuing fertility of the land and increases the nutrient value and flavor of the food grown in it, as we discussed in chapter one.

> Soil is one of our nation's most valuable resources and it needs to be treated well or we risk losing it. Soil conservation and management have been a priority on our farm for many, many years. In our peach orchard, we have used mulches and natural soil amendments that help keep the trees healthy, so the trees can take up maximum sugars into their fruit. Our customers notice that our peaches taste better and come back year after year. Paying close attention to soil condition is not only better for the environment but also produces more nutritious and tasty food.
>
> *~Walter S. is a mostly retired farmer who continues to tend his orchard. He started incorporating natural methods on his 40-acre farm long before "sustainable agriculture" and "organic farming" became popular.*

The World Resources Institute estimates that the average farm would show a $29 per acre *loss* if the true costs of soil loss, water contamination, and other environmental degradation were taken into account.[19] Soil loss can happen very quickly compared to the time it takes to replace topsoil, which is anywhere from 20 to 1000 years. In the past 200 years, the United States has lost a third of our cropland topsoil.[20] To prevent these losses, farmers need to replace topsoil continually by adding organic matter in the form of manure, cover crops, mulches, etc.

Here again, remember that "locally grown" does not necessarily mean that good farming practices are being used. However, when you deal directly with the grower, you can verify for yourself whether their farming practices are in line with your values—something that is difficult to do when the grower lives 1500 miles away.

---

19   Vasilikiotis, Christos, Ph.D. "Can Organic Farming Feed the World?" University of California, Berkeley, www.cnr.berkeley.edu/~christos/articles/cv_organic_farming.html.

20   "Food and the Environment," www.foodroutes.org/hottopic.jsp?id=3.

JUST FOOD

Many people choose to eat locally for social justice reasons. Choosing locally and sustainably grown foods can be a way to align ourselves with the interests of the poor and support more equitable systems of food production. Not only do the poor bear the burden of scarcity when we overuse the world's limited resources, but they disproportionately suffer from the environmental side effects—problems like toxic waste, contaminated water supplies, pesticide poisoning, etc. Eating simply (locally, seasonally, and lower on the food chain) requires less of the earth's finite resources than the standard American diet, and supports a network of small farms rather than a chain of giant agribusinesses.

The anonymity of supermarket food makes it difficult to know anything about the working conditions of its producers. Did migrant workers produce it? Dispossessed tenant farmers? Slave or child labor? Were the farm workers exposed to harmful chemicals or unsafe working conditions? Were they compensated fairly? By buying local, you can find out the answers to these questions and ensure that the growers who raised your dinner were treated well.

We all have items that are not available in our locales, but that are difficult to give up. Coffee, chocolate, and tea are commonly cited examples. Unfortunately, many growers of these products are poorly paid and mistreated. Their desperate circumstances (and the greed of some multinational corporations) can lead to environmental damage as well. One way to help alleviate such problems is to buy fairly traded items. Fair trade certification ensures fair price, fair labor conditions, environmental sustainability, and direct trade. You can read more at the Fair Trade Certified website, www.transfairusa.org. Buying fairly traded items is perhaps the closest you can come to the spirit of buying local in terms of social justice around the globe.

Social justice is not just an issue for people halfway around the world; many needy people among us can benefit from a network of local growers. Programs like "Plant a Row for the Hungry" are on the increase, and some farmers contribute excess produce to local food banks. One family we interviewed gets permission from small growers near them to glean the end-of-season vegetables from their fields, and then distributes them to needy families. This family, like many other gardeners, enjoys sharing the abundance of their own garden with neighbors and friends. Imagine the impact on world hunger that millions of generous gardeners and farmers could have!

Overall, by beginning to shift our diet towards locally grown, seasonal foods, we have found a greater joy in growing, purchasing, cooking, and eating our food. I really got into this full swing after our summer trip to Kenya in 2006, where I was confronted daily with issues of hunger, poverty, and scarcity. Coming home, I was confronted daily with abundance and excess, a cultural addiction to convenience and entitlement. I longed for some way to channel my uncertainty and frustration over what I saw and heard in Kenya (and other developing countries I have visited) into some small step towards a healthier, more just world. I had purchased a *Simply in Season* cookbook earlier that year, but hadn't really used it much. My husband and I started digging into it more and learning more about how our food choices affect the broader world. Though not directly affecting the people and places I visited in Kenya, I felt shifting our meals toward fresh, wholesome vegetables and fruits was contributing in a small way toward making the world livable for all of us.

I think eating seasonally has deepened my spirituality—I have become more in touch with the rhythms of the natural world and disciplined myself not to expect to get what I want whenever I want it (i.e., strawberries in January). Refraining from purchasing some foods at certain times of the year helps me to remember that much of the world lives constantly with very little. What has become an expected way of eating for many of us in the United States is actually very unusual worldwide, and continuing to live with the consumption and excess that we do is hurting Creation.

I now often remember to think of those in developing countries as I say a prayer before meals. Moreover, I think we also treasure the treats more than we used to—strawberries in June, tomatoes in September, pumpkin seeds in November—we savor them! (It is probably even a shift to consider fruits and vegetables a treat...they used to be more of a burden, something "good for you" that you have to add to your diet.) Experiencing delight and gratefulness for these little miracles has deepened my connection to God and helped me feel more joyful and appreciative.

~Laura S. and her husband currently live in a Cleveland, OH suburb. She is a social worker and her husband is in medical school. A shady backyard prompted them to do their gardening at a community garden a block away where they have gleaned much wisdom from seasoned gardeners.

SPIRITUALITY

Mindful eating is a spiritual act or discipline for many people. They feel a connection to God as they eat in a way that honors and protects Creation. Some speak of a calling to care for the earth and its inhabitants—plant, animal, and human. Others note a deepening awareness of the rhythms of the natural world as they learn to eat more seasonally, and an increased appreciation for the earth's bounty and variety. In our survey, both farmers and eaters noted this connection. Ron and Mary M. of Strawberry Hill Farm wrote, "Another benefit of farming on a small scale and using more hand labor is the more intimate connection to the earth and to its Creator. There is definitely a spiritual and even holy element to working with soil, plants, and animals." The Amish are also well known for their choice to limit technology in order to keep their farms small and their communities tight. *Farming Magazine*, edited by Amish farmer and author David Kline, is a valuable resource for anyone interested in learning to farm on a small scale and to appreciate the rhythms of the natural world.

Christians are not alone in recognizing a spiritual element to their food and certainly not the first to do so. Native Americans and other traditional cultures have long celebrated and recognized a spiritual connection with both the earth and its Creator. By making our food supply anonymous, and by treating animals and plants as simply production units rather than as living things, industrial farming separates us from the sense of reverence and gratitude that we naturally feel in response to the earth's bounteous gifts.

Before making a choice about consuming something, including food, I often ask myself if this would be a loving action toward my neighbor. I think of a "neighbor" as any human being, with the realization that we are living in a global community. Most often I figure buying locally is the most beneficial for all my global neighbors.

Benefits include relationships with families and farmers around us. Our consciousness is awakened and aware of how our actions affect those around us. There is a sense that by supporting our neighbors and God's planet in this way we are making a choice to do the right thing. Living this way helps us to remember that we are not the only humans on the planet and our actions can harm or help others.

~Sommer D. is the mother of three young children. She raises vegetables, flowers, and chickens in her front yard and her husband is gradually transforming the rest of the yard into a prairie garden to reduce the need for mowing.

SAVE A FARMER: BUY LOCAL

When it comes to shopping, most of us think in terms of low prices, selection, and brand name appeal. And no wonder—advertisers continually bombard us with messages that reinforce this way of thinking. However, looking more carefully and connecting the dots between our shopping habits and the health of our towns will show that the way we spend our money determines the fate of our communities. As we take our business farther and farther from home, we act against our own local economies. Food is the primary focus of this book, but these principles apply to a broader range of goods and services as well.

ECONOMIC BENEFITS TO THE LOCAL ECONOMY

The evidence is piling up: spending money at local businesses really does pay off. Below are some recent findings from all over the United States:

If every **Michigan** family bought just $10/week of Michigan produce, it would keep $1.9 billion annually from leaving the state, generate almost 2000 new jobs, and increase farm income as much as 16%.[21]

---

21 Marshall, Jane, "'Buy Local' mindset could boost state's economy," *The Vegetable Growers News*, March 2008. (Michigan Land Use Institute study "Eat Fresh and Grow Jobs")

$1 billion is spent in food dollars in the 7-county area that includes Cleveland, **Ohio**, but only 1% is produced locally. Increasing that to just 10% would add $700 million to local agricultural income.[22]

In **Maine**, switching just 1% of food purchases to local foods would translate into a 5% increase in farmers' incomes. A $10 weekly purchase of local foods by Maine residents would invest $100,000,000 back into the local economy each growing season, according to the Maine Organic Farmers and Gardeners Association (MOFGA). [23]

> The simple act of buying locally contributes to creating a greater sense of community. I have gained a greater appreciation for the local character of my community. The simple act of buying local food has also led me to commit to other local choices—the bakery, local artisans, the local bank, and the small theater downtown. These small investments are dollars poured back into the community. Together they help sustain a strong local economy. I cannot think of a better way to help preserve diversity and local character—an antidote to the homogenous formula of super-sized supermarkets, restaurant chains, and department stores that dictate our choices and breed cultural ennui.
>
> *~Monique T. is a local foods aficionado both at her own table and in the catering business she ran for several seasons. The dramatic use of herbs and edible flowers are some of her trademarks in showcasing the season's best.*

BENEFITS ABROAD

As we mentioned earlier, buying fairly traded items is one way to ensure that the workers who produced those items are treated well and compensated fairly for their labor, and to support sustainable production practices. Fair Trade is a good option for purchasing special items that are not grown locally; however, because of the environmental consequences of long-distance transport, the most sustainable option is still to purchase locally made or grown items when possible.

---

22   Cuyahoga Valley Countryside Conservancy, http://www.cvcountryside.org/food/why-buy-local.php

23   "Buy Local Challenge," www.foodroutes.org/buy-local-challenge.jsp.

What began as simply a convenient (my primary local food source is a very good friend of mine!) way to get very fresh vegetables, meats, and eggs has turned into an intentional effort to eat locally whatever possible. Our efforts now include milk and yogurt as well. I am also much more aware of eating foods that are in season, and avoiding buying foods that must be shipped in from faraway places. Basically, I try to plan my menus around the foods that are available locally (I'm far from being 100% on this, but I'm better than I used to be), and attempt to make my own foods from scratch to avoid processed/prepared foods whenever possible.

I admit that I mostly have made my choices because it benefits my family directly, and my friends the farmers directly. Occasionally I also pat myself on the back for doing something that is good for the environment or for global trade or something like that. I get depressed when I think about what a difference we could make in the world if everyone would choose to eat just one thing a week that is produced locally, and so I try to remind myself that it's the little steps that count.

~Amy G. is a violinist and the mother of four who also creates custom baby slings for appreciative mothers. Her small backyard is flanked with berry bushes and garden beds. She enjoys shopping at local markets.

ECONOMIC INDEPENDENCE

Agriculture in this country has become more and more "vertically integrated;" that is, consolidated into the hands of a few powerful agribusinesses, leaving farmers as essentially employees of those companies. Grain farmers may find that one large company sells them seed and chemicals, owns the grain elevator, and sets the price it will pay. Poultry growers contract with agribusinesses that provide chicks, feed, and slaughter facilities. Many find themselves trapped in a never-ending cycle of debt that forces them to raise more and more animals in order to pay off their expensive buildings. Cattle and hog farmers are in the same boat. Eric Schlosser notes that four meatpacking companies controlled 21% of the beef market in 1970. This has risen to nearly 85% today.[24] Unfortunately, growers under

---

24   Schlosser, Eric, "Cheap Food Nation," *Sierra*, Nov/Dec 2006.

contract to these large integrated producers add little to the local economy, hauling feed in and animals out of the area to their own processing facilities. Small, independent farms may find themselves excluded from markets, slaughter facilities, etc. as these mega-corporations prefer to contract with their own growers.

The reality for many farmers is that one spouse needs to work full-time off the farm to help pay the bills and provide an affordable healthcare plan. Many farmers long to devote their full-time attention to their passion but can't afford to.

On the bright side, however, the growing consumer interest in local and sustainably grown foods is benefiting some small farms. Many are coming up with creative ways of marketing and advertising their products. Green Field Farms is a case in point, an innovative cooperative of Amish farmers who banded together to market their organically grown eggs, milk, cheese, and produce under the Green Fields label in an effort to keep their families on the land. Other farmers have begun to direct market their products in order to capture more of the profits. The Cuyahoga Valley Countryside Conservancy reports that farmers receive only 9¢ of each dollar spent in conventional markets but 80-90¢ of each dollar when they sell their products through a farmers' market or CSA.[25]

To make direct marketing work for farmers, we need to buy their products. Adam H., an Amish farmer who raises produce and pastured meats, commented, "The day after we moved to our farm, a local lady stopped by to tell us that she and some of her friends would like to start buying meats and produce from us. She has been a supportive customer and we actually named our first Jersey cow after her! We also had people just the opposite. They stopped in for chicken and when they heard the price, they almost fell over and said they can get it at Kroger's for half that."

The local foods movement has also opened up a new agribusiness niche: the mobile slaughter plant. These small slaughter facilities are designed for small farmers and ranchers to process their own meat on the farm in an inspected facility. This allows them to legally market their meat to restaurants, farmers' markets, etc. The USDA is now promoting these plants and even providing loans to help finance them.

---

25   "Why Go Local?" Cuyahoga Valley Countryside Conservancy, http://www. cvcountryside.org/food/why-buy-local.php.

COMMUNITY

We find that supporting our local economy strengthens our connections to the community and our sense of place in it; a benefit that is unquantifiable but valuable nonetheless. And we find that this local life is a joyful thing. At the Geiser farm, we enjoy relating to our customers. As people regularly show up at the farm for eggs, veggies, flowers, etc., we connect with their lives. Small conversations take place during the exchange and we learn about their grandchildren, deaths in the family, or vacation plans. Folks are often curious about events on the farm and in our family. When I am aware of something significant happening in their lives, I can quickly add a small bouquet to their purchase to let them know that I care. I had a small bouquet ready for a customer in memory of her special aunt who just passed away and I quickly gathered a handful of mini pink zinnias for another customer on the day she shared the news of her pregnancy (she did have a girl!).

Elementary teacher Joni F. observed, "I think right now we live in a world of individualism. There is a lack of community. People have learned to take care of themselves and do everything on their own. If people could see and experience the joy of living in community, where we help each other, support each other, and look out for the needs of our neighbors, I think they would take a lot of pleasure in knowing that by buying locally grown foods, they are supporting someone in their community."

Studies show that people have ten times more conversations at farmers' markets than they do at supermarkets.[26] Apparently, the very nature of the market lends itself to relationship. Small farms and businesses cannot always compete on price, but they usually offer stellar service and go out of their way to be helpful.

> I love to talk with the farmers at the farmers' market each week. Sometimes my children wake early and come with me to meet the folks who grow their food. When we thank God for the food before a meal, we can name the people who helped bring the food to our table. Always in my mind are

---

26   Halweil, Brian, *Eat Here: Homegrown Pleasures in a Global Supermarket* (W.W. Norton & Co.: 2004) 10.

the long-term effects of my local purchases. I've heard that economists have agreed that the best thing people can do to reduce carbon emissions is to eat locally. When I grow my own food and buy food from my neighbors here in the Shenandoah Valley, I am helping save the world!

I really view this as our family's main political action, as well as our investment portfolio, the family health insurance plan, and a global awareness program. It feels like my "calling," my gift to my family and community, the earth, and all creatures. I believe deeply that God made a wonderful and marvelous universe and asks us to care for this, our home.

~Kris S.Z. is a musician and mother of two. She home educates her children and manages to grow an astonishing quantity of food in a small patch of land behind her apartment. Kris is a dedicated farmers' market shopper and participates in a food co-op as well.

As local artisans are encouraged to develop their craft, whether it be building furniture from native wood or creating a signature salsa, perhaps each region will redevelop its own unique flavor. Imagine how much more interesting it would be to travel the countryside and discover each community's specialties than to travel the world and eat from the same menu at every McDonald's.

Living and eating locally takes a little extra effort, but has big payoffs for our local economies, environments, and communities. Supporting local farms and businesses is a simple but effective way to improve your own local economy and to strengthen relationships at the same time. As you plan your next shopping trip, whether for soap, gifts, or a gallon of milk, don't forget to connect the dots, and to consider how your purchases will influence the future of your community. As we realize the power we have to shape the environment, the soil, social issues, our spirituality, and more at the dinner table, our meals become more complicated, but also more fulfilling. We truly can change the world by voting with our forks.

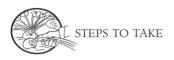 STEPS TO TAKE

1. Figure out your own food miles. Take an average meal and calculate how far the ingredients have traveled. Does it fit the 1500-mile average? How could you reduce your average?

2. Find a way to replace one item in your pantry with a local or fairly traded item. Coffee and chocolate are an easy place to start, as fairly traded versions of these foods are available in many stores and by mail order (try www.equalexchange.com or www.justcoffee.com, for starters, or enter "fair trade" or "equal exchange" in a search engine). Even better, replace an occasional cup of coffee with a local tea or other beverage.

3. Consider offering a few words of thankfulness at each meal to cultivate a spirit of mindfulness and appreciation for the earth's bounty and those who work the soil.

4. Engage a local farmer in conversation about how people's food choices affect their family.

 RESOURCES

1. *The Small-Mart Revolution: How Local Businesses Are Beating the Global Competition* by Michael H. Shuman

2. *Big-Box Swindle: The True Cost of Mega-Retailers and the Fight for America's Independent Businesses* by Stacy Mitchell

3. *The Omnivore's Dilemma* by Michael Pollan

4. *Serve God, Save the Planet* by J. Matthew Sleeth

5. *Scratching the Woodchuck* and *Great Possessions* by David Kline

6. *The Future of Food* DVD by Deborah Koons Garcia

7. *Farming Magazine*, www.farmingmagazine.net (P.O. Box 85, Mt. Hope, OH 44660)

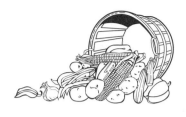

CHAPTER 3

Eating with the Seasons

*Live in each season as it passes, breathe the air, drink the drink, taste the fruit,
and resign yourself to the influence of each.*
- Henry David Thoreau

One of the basics of eating locally is learning to eat in season. You may or may not be aware that strawberries are a late spring delicacy, that local sweet corn won't appear naturally until mid-summer, and that you should look for the best sweet potatoes in fall. Unlike our ancestors, not everyone today has a clear sense of what is in season, thanks to modern supermarkets that foster the illusion that everything is available year-round. Learning to eat with the seasons is a skill that needs to be relearned. It will benefit your taste buds, your pocketbook, your health, and your local economy.

Since seasonality varies by region, observing what is available at farmers' markets and roadside stands is a first step in discovering the seasonal schedule for your area. Joni F. finds a seasonal cookbook helpful in determining what foods are in season. "I have loved using the *Simply in Season* cookbook that we received as a wedding gift because I wasn't necessarily aware of all the foods that are in season during a particular time. It helps me to know what to look for and what will be best during that time," she says.

Included in the back of this book is Appendix C, which lists when basic produce is available throughout the year. You might want to post a copy of this page on your refrigerator or in a cupboard to help you get started. Later in the book, we will discuss more about where to find local foods in your area, how you can grow your own, and what to do in the off-season.

BENEFITS OF EATING SEASONALLY

Eating with the seasons benefits both farmers and consumers. For farmers, the ability to sell freshly harvested produce means they don't have to install costly storage systems. This translates into lower costs for the consumer during peak seasons for most fruits and vegetables. The fluctuation in prices of items like tomatoes or green beans at the farmers' market will quickly tell you when peak season hits and farmers are trying to move products at lower prices rather than tossing them in the compost pile.

Amazingly, each season can also give our bodies what we need for our climate. The dark leafy greens of spring act as cleansing agents to rid our bodies of winter toxins. Summer provides juicy melons and tomatoes to help keep us hydrated in sweltering conditions while the dense starchy root vegetables of fall allow us to store up energy for winter.

Disciplining oneself to follow the seasons also creates a renewed sense of celebration. Eating freshly picked produce at the peak of flavor is ambrosia to the taste buds, especially after waiting for it so long. Chefs know this secret of good taste and it is hard to find a high-end restaurant that doesn't offer a seasonal menu. Eating seasonally keeps our sense of taste invigorated and truly offers cause for celebration when you eat the first meal of sweet corn or sample a few of the earliest blueberries.

SQUASH OVERLOAD

After consuming our fill of the current season's produce, we tend to get a bit weary of it. "Zucchini *again?*" the children complain. But it's not long before the next food comes into its season of abundance. Kelly S.'s family has built a family tradition around seasonal produce. "One of our favorite meals is fresh tomatoes on toast with mayonnaise, fresh cantaloupe, and fresh cucumbers in sour cream," she says. "We look forward every year to the time we can have that meal almost weekly until the season is done."

When the Amstutz family first began to make an intentional effort to eat seasonal, locally grown foods, we were surprised to find ourselves actually eating a larger variety of foods than before—just not all at once. We started buying odd sorts of squash, trying parsnips and turnips and other vegetables that would never previously have merited a second glance, and found that we actually liked some of the new foods. (Though we still don't like turnips!) There's a good chance you'll discover some new favorites too. We discovered that there are indeed things to eat year-round in Ohio—we just had to learn to notice them.

Still, while it can be done, most people have trouble limiting themselves completely to local produce, unless they live in a warm climate. Besides, even those fortunate folks might get a hankering for some maple syrup or cherries once in awhile. There's nothing wrong with indulging in a few non-local specialties. However, when choosing those luxury produce items, it is still wise to learn when they are in season wherever they are grown and to purchase them when they are plentiful, flavorful, and inexpensive. Even oranges, mangoes, and pineapples have a peak season. You can usually figure out when it is by paying attention to price, flavor, and availability in the grocery store, or by looking up the information in a cookbook or on the web.

SPRING FEVER

The earliest taste of spring comes in the form of aromatic maple syrup boiled down from the sap of trees just waking from their long winter's nap. Fresh syrup is a delicious way to kick off the growing season and one food cooperative in our area even bottles and sells maple sap distillate as a healthful drink. The next fresh tastes of spring are the salad greens, scallions, radishes, wild ramps, asparagus, and rhubarb. Folk wisdom names some of the earliest greens of spring—dandelion greens and stinging nettle shoots— as effective spring tonics for rejuvenating our systems. Even the chickens and cows on pasture benefit from spring's lush growth of grass, causing milk and egg production to increase.

Admittedly, spring produce can be heavy on the green and slim on variety, leaving us craving the next act after weeks of giant salads. Spring's finale consists of peas and a welcome burst of color in the form of strawberries. Eating the first vine-ripened strawberry of the season is definitely one of those times when food evokes a celebration. Susan M.L., whose children are now young adults, reminisced about their family strawberry traditions. "Strawberries are precious to our

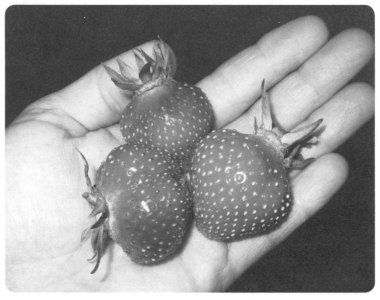

Strawberries are one of the first fruity pleasures of the year. Forgoing long-distance berries in favor of local, vine-ripened ones makes them a treat to savor when strawberry season finally arrives.

family because we don't eat them out of season," she said. "The ones from California may be huge, but they lack taste and juice. We wait until our own berries are ripe, bring the first ones in, and carefully share them. This tradition matters to our children; our daughter turns down any strawberries out-of-season so that first taste can be anticipated and savored."

SUMMER TREATS

As temperatures rise, lettuce turns bitter, radishes get pithy, spinach begins to bolt, and thankfully, the summer vegetables are starting to come onstage. New potatoes, green beans, zucchini, and an early taste of sweet corn and tomatoes now make an appearance on our plates. Strawberry season melts into raspberries, then blueberries and blackberries and other fruits like peaches and pears start bearing. Summer is when farmers' markets are in their glory with additional vendors and tables heaped with a colorful abundance of produce. Now is the time to eat entire meals of melons or sweet corn and to lavish fresh herbs like basil in all of your cooking. For meat connoisseurs, the first pastured chickens, raised outdoors on fresh grass, are ready for butchering and often will be available until the snow flies.

At times, summer may also bring drought or untimely hailstorms, which can be hard on crops. Learning to be understanding of what the farmer is facing and sometimes needing to accept zucchini pockmarked by last week's hailstorm is part of learning to eat with the seasons.

AUTUMN HARVEST

Many summer crops will continue producing until the first frost hits. Meanwhile, fall crops have made their debut as cooler weather comes around. Winter squashes and root crops like beets, carrots, and turnips join with apples to bring new flavors to our table. Salad greens return for an encore performance and some crops like cabbage, broccoli, and Brussels sprouts will actually develop more sweetness after exposure to frost. We instinctively start eating more hearty soups and stews to warm ourselves, accompanied by pumpkins and apple cider. Many farmers will be taking animals to the butcher this time of year rather than feeding them over the winter, so it may be a good time to purchase meats. Egg customers need to be patient while hens undergo a molt and slow their production.

WINTER WONDERS

In colder climates, winter is a more challenging time to find local foods. Except for a few hardy greens that can be grown in greenhouses or cold frames, there is little fresh produce from the field or garden available. There are still local foods around, however, if you know where to look.

Meats, milk, and eggs are generally available year-round, though they may be less plentiful this time of year. Grains are often available through the winter also because they are easily stored. Many autumn vegetables can be kept in a cool place through much of the winter, so foods like apples, cabbage, onions, garlic, squash, carrots, etc. can still be eaten if you plan ahead. Food preservation—canning, freezing, or dehydrating—is another good way to ensure a steady supply of local foods even through the winter.

Because winter is such a tough time for the locavore, we have expanded more fully on this topic later in this book. See chapter nine for ideas on how you can squirrel away foods for the lean months.

CONCLUSION

This is only a brief introduction to the produce available in each season; you will discover many more possibilities as you start searching for local foods in your area. As you learn to eat seasonally, it may at times feel like a sacrifice. Bypassing peppers or fresh berries from another hemisphere and learning to wait until they come into season in your area takes some self-discipline and planning. Sometimes this will mean adjusting your menu plan to accommodate what is available; other times it will mean using a home-frozen or canned version while you wait on the next season to roll around. We believe that the celebration of fresh tastes will make your sacrifice worthwhile.

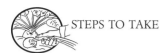 STEPS TO TAKE

1. Set a goal of cooking a meal once a week with a seasonal ingredient.

2. Cut out or copy the chart at the end of this book and stick it on your refrigerator.

3. Find out what's in season this month in your area. Check with your local extension office. Search out one local item to substitute for what you normally buy. Try a taste test to see if your friends or family can taste the difference.

 RESOURCES

1. *Simply in Season (World Community Cookbook)* by Mary Beth Lind and Cathleen Hockman-Wert.

2. *From Asparagus to Zucchini: A Guide to Cooking Farm-Fresh Seasonal Produce* by the Madison Area Community Supported Agriculture Coalition.

SEASONAL MENU IDEAS

The year our family began in earnest to eat locally and seasonally, I kept a journal of our menus and experiences. The following menus come from those journal entries. The majority of these ingredients were either homegrown or purchased from nearby farmers.

SPRING

Polish sausage
Homemade French fries
Garden salad
Rhubarb Crunch

Velvety spring soup (spinach and onions, leeks
and potatoes)
Garden salad with sugar snap peas, radishes, onions,
and hard-boiled eggs

Creamed eggs over homemade biscuits
Garden salad
Cherries (frozen)

Grilled chicken
Ohio potatoes
Garden salad with radishes, onions, chive flowers,
and eggs
Homemade applesauce

SUMMER

Creamed turkey over noodles
Garden salad
Lemon thyme bread
Local peaches

Grilled eggplant burgers
Grilled zucchini slices
Tomato, pepper, and mushroom kebabs
Locally made noodles
Grilled nectarine halves

Scalloped potatoes with ham
Acorn squash
Apple Crisp

Crockpot Corn Chowder
Tomatoes
Edamame
Sliced cucumbers

FALL

Ratatouille (eggplant, peppers, summer squash, and tomatoes) over spaghetti noodles
Broccoli salad

Roasted chicken
Baked sweet potatoes
Homemade coleslaw

Tomato soup
Grilled cheese sandwiches
Spinach salad topped with eggs

Gingery Squash Soup
Cinnamon-topped Oatmeal Muffins
Salad

WINTER

Potato, leek, and kale soup
Salad
Homemade bread and jam

Lemon herb chicken
Ohio potatoes (baked)
Salad
Apple Crisp

Shredded barbecued beef sandwiches
Cooked carrots
Potato wedges
Ice cream

Lentil-Beef Skillet
Savory Kale
Homemade oatmeal bread

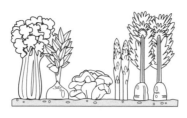

CHAPTER 4

Finding Local Foods

W hen I (Lisa) was about five years old, my aunt and uncle invited my family to a big treasure hunt. Adults and children alike scoured the house and yard for hidden clues, each of which led to the next clue. I've forgotten what the ultimate treasure was, but I do remember the thrill of the hunt. It's a thrill I still get to experience now and then in my quest to find locally grown foods—the satisfaction of finding a source of local oatmeal, a new farmers' market, or a farm stand off the beaten path.

Local, organic carrots or free-range eggs never seem to be advertised on television (though advertisers are intent on making sure we recognize all 300 brands of neon-colored, sugarcoated cereal) and no glossy flyers ever appear in our mailboxes to inform us when asparagus is in season. It takes a little detective work to track down local foods, but one clue leads to the next, as in any good treasure hunt. The treasure, of course, is fresh, delicious produce, meats, cheeses, etc. There are many farms, markets, auctions, and even supermarkets where you can discover wonderful local foods, and they may even be as close as your backyard.

FARMERS' MARKETS

The number of farmers' markets in the United States has skyrocketed in recent years, and their popularity continues to increase as interest in local foods grows. If you are fortunate enough to live near one, a farmers' market is an excellent place to purchase local items directly from the producer. Most markets are open once a week for a several-hour time slot, often in a downtown location. Farmers' market shopping is much simpler than driving out to each farm to pick up individual purchases. Market sizes can vary from just a handful of vendors to a hundred or more offering a wide variety of produce, meats, and cottage industry creations.

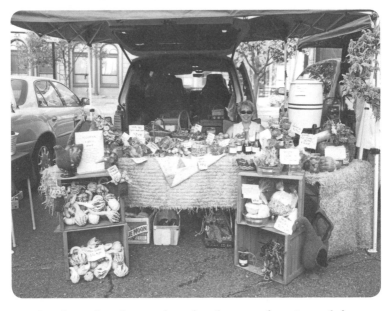

At a farmers' market, you have the advantage of meeting each farmer face-to-face. A stroll through the market offers a glimpse at the uniqueness of each farm and an abundance of fresh, seasonal offerings.

Ruth C. is a frequent shopper at the weekly Wooster farmers' market. She says, "I go to the farmers' market every Saturday for fresh and unusual items such as locally grown Lion's Mane mushrooms, fresh bread, and fruits (strawberries, blueberries, and blackberries) which I do not grow myself. Sweet corn season is fabulous due to our local farmers who make the trip into town to sell their produce. My Turkish friend is there selling her marvelous stuffed grape leaves, hummus, and tabouleh; she also makes beautiful jewelry and shawls. There is wonderful fellowship, banjo music, free kittens, locally grown beef, coffee shops close by, and the beautiful atmosphere of our lovely downtown. I like watching people leave with bouquets of fresh flowers and French bread peeking out of their own 'green' grocery bags. Parents with their children in strollers and dogs on leashes only add to the feeling that we live in a great community! It is such fun to catch up with old friends and meet new ones!"

Farmers' market shopping is serendipitous—you never quite know what you'll find. It can be frustrating if you're hunting for a specific item, but the unexpectedness of this kind of shopping is part of the fun of it too. Some markets offer live musical entertainment that adds to the atmosphere. In cooler climates, markets may move indoors for the winter months but most run only during the growing season (June to October).

For the best selection at the farmers' market, shop early, before things are sold out—popular items like strawberries, sweet corn, and tomatoes often sell out quickly, particularly at the beginning of the season. On the other hand, you may be able to score some bargains at the end of the day, when farmers would rather make a deal than haul their goods back home again. It's a good idea to scan all the booths first, noting what's available and checking the prices, then decide where to make your purchases. Be sure to do your part for the environment—bring along your market bag!

Monique T., a local caterer, is able to source many of the ingredients for her gourmet meals at the market. "I shop at our local farmers' market throughout the season and collaborate with a local grower in planning seasonal offerings for my 'mostly organic' & seasonal vegetarian meal service," she explains. "I extend the local foods season well into November by driving to a few farms that have potatoes, apples, cider, honey, maple syrup, squash, and pumpkin available after the market season is over."

OUR STORY (LISA)

My husband and I are both the first generation to grow up off the farm—our grandparents were corn, grass seed, and dairy farmers. So perhaps it is in our blood. Since we didn't inherit any farmland, though, we've had to content ourselves with a six-acre homestead, and my husband continues his day job while I freelance from home. We provide ourselves with most of our own meat, eggs, goat milk, honey, fruits, and vegetables and occasionally have extras to sell directly or at the farmers' market.

Some days I wonder why we put ourselves through this, like the day I found myself chasing our three pigs down the road in a downpour, or the day the children's favorite goat died. There is little profit in what we do, and there is always, always work to be done and not enough time at the end of the day to do it all.

But it is worth it to know where our food is coming from and that our animals are treated humanely—the chickens get to dust-bathe and scratch for bugs, the pigs root and wallow, etc. We know that our fruits and vegetables have not been sprayed with any toxic chemicals, that our meat is hormone and antibiotic-free, and that our soil is growing more and more nutrient-rich every year as we pile on manure, leaves, and cover crops.

We have the satisfaction of watching our children learn to garden and care for their own animals. They also get to ride goats, dabble in the creek, and build tunnels among the hay bales in the barn. They are learning to work alongside us, whether the task is shoveling out the barn, setting up a farmers' market stand, or making pickles.

Best of all, we have the satisfaction of knowing that we will someday leave this piece of land in better condition than we found it—more fertile and more beautiful, with more trees, flowers, and wildlife habitat. As suburban sprawl creeps closer and closer, this one piece of land, at least, will be protected and preserved for the next generation.

SUPERMARKET STRATEGIES

The most convenient way to begin eating locally is simply to look for locally grown or produced items at your grocery store. Check labels carefully—in addition to local produce, meat, and dairy, you may be able to find local condiments such as mustards, salsas, or salad dressings, baked goods, pastas, etc.

If you can't find much, or if items are not well labeled, encourage your grocery store manager to buy more regional produce and label it as such. Let them know it is important to you as a customer. Andrea G., a musician and mother of five, uses this strategy. "I try to shop at our locally owned grocery store instead of large chain stores, and watch for produce that is specifically marked as locally grown. I take the time to tell the produce manager I appreciate when they carry these kinds of items."

Small, regional grocery stores may be the most receptive to these suggestions, though some larger chains are beginning to source more of their produce locally and clearly label it as such in response to consumer demand. Interestingly, country-of-origin labeling (COOL) for beef, lamb, pork, fish, perishable agricultural commodities, and peanuts was signed into law with the 2002 Farm Bill. However, Congress delayed implementing the law until 2009, when it went into effect with some notable exceptions.[28]

In this region, we have a number of small enterprises that supply local supermarkets with their products along with a dairy, poultry processor, and potato farm that produce on a commercial scale but have the reputation of treating their employees well and producing quality products. Learning to identify local labels and purchasing them regularly will help to prevent the corporate giants from gobbling up their shelf space. In our experience, supporting a locally owned grocery store is worth the few extra dollars it may cost. These stores tend to stock more local products than the chain stores and give back to the community in many ways. In addition, locally owned stores are often more willing to accommodate customer requests.

Buehler's is a family-owned chain of grocery stores in northeast Ohio. They are committed to buying from Ohio businesses and intentional in labeling produce as "local." Produce buyer Dave Graf buys directly from many Ohio farms and travels semiweekly to an area produce auction where he purchases two to six semi loads of locally grown vegetables for the thirteen regional Buehler's stores. "It is a good situation for both us and the growers," Dave said. "We can work together with the growers on suggesting varieties and best packing practices, and staggering availability. Buying direct from the farmer lowers freight costs and also benefits the consumer by bringing down the cost."

28   USDA Agricultural Marketing Service: Country of Origin Labeling. www.ams. usda.gov/AMSv1.0/cool.

When searching for locally grown or produced items at the supermarket, be careful—labels can be misleading at times. Just because a food is "packed by" a local company, for instance, doesn't mean it was actually grown or produced locally. You should probably be suspicious if a food is labeled as local but isn't in season where you live—unless it's grown in a greenhouse, it's probably "greenwashing."

"Greenwashing" is when companies try to appear more environmentally friendly than they really are. For more examples, see www.greenwashing.net.

OTHER KINDS OF STORES

Nontraditional grocery stores are another good avenue for finding local products. Small, family-owned stores specializing in local products are popping up in many places. One store we visited offered local meats, dairy, eggs, grains, and produce in season along with the unique feature of hand-dipped ice cream (from a local dairy) to serve hot and hungry bikers from a nearby bike path. Their goal is to be a connection for consumers and farmers and to offer quality products that are good for people's health, spirituality, and the community. Many customers choose to patronize their store instead of larger natural food chains because they like the personal attention that is given. According to its founder, the store purchases only products produced in the United States and specifically in Ohio when possible. Several customers who produce things like handmade soap, brooms and essential oils have added their products to the store's shelves as well.

Many communities also have co-ops and health food or bulk food stores, which sometimes carry local items. Because things are often packaged in bulk and not clearly labeled, you may need to ask a clerk to find out where the food came from. Whole Foods has jumped on the local foods bandwagon as well, and is making a considerable effort to carry some local products in each of their stores.[29]

29　"Locally Grown: The Whole Foods Promise." http.//www.wholefoodsmarket.com/products/locally-grown/index.php.

DIRECT FROM THE FARM

If you're willing to go the extra mile to buy directly from a farmer, you have a number of options. The simplest of these is the farm store or roadside stand. Usually you'll spot a sign by the side of the road advertising available items. This option is hit-or-miss, but it is possible to find some bargains, with no commitment required on your part. You may want to call ahead to see what's available, or join the farm's mailing list.

I (Karen) needed sweet corn for a family gathering and was headed to a well-stocked farm stand five miles away. Two miles down the road I noticed a hand-lettered sign for sweet corn and, being conscious of gas prices, decided to give it a try. I found a small farm building with a neat display of extra veggies. A 12-year-old boy who had helped pick the corn that morning recognized me from an event in town and very politely helped me with my purchase. The next time I need sweet corn, I'll try this farm first. In the future, gas prices may force all of us to discover the treasures our neighbors have to offer and connect us to our communities in unexpected ways.

Pick-your-own farms are popular in some areas, and allow customers to harvest their own fruit, berries, or vegetables. Since the farmer does not need to cover the labor costs of harvesting, prices are usually lower. You provide the quality control, eliminating that disappointing experience of finding squishy berries at the bottom of the basket or one rotten apple in the bag. Pick-your-owns are a great, hands-on way to teach children about where their food comes from and make fun family outings. (www.pickyourown.org lists pick-your-own farms by state.)

There are a growing number of produce auctions, particularly in areas with a high concentration of Amish farms, which offer bulk quantities of produce to the highest bidder. If you happen to live near a produce auction, you can score great bargains with a little luck and patience. Most things will be in large lots, which are great for canning or freezing but will be more than the average family can consume fresh. Just be vigilant and make sure you know what you're getting, as items may not be well labeled and prices can vary wildly according to season and demand. (One family specifically plans to buy their sweet corn for freezing just before Labor Day weekend, when grocery stores are buying less due to the holiday and prices tend to be lower.) As at any auction, the principle of *caveat emptor* applies: buyer beware!

ORDERING FROM THE FARM

Many farmers take advance orders for larger items like chickens or a side of beef. Signing up for a farm newsletter is a good way to find out about these offers, and some farms now have websites.

If you want to ensure a steady stream of fresh foods, consider signing up for a CSA (Community Supported Agriculture) share, where you purchase a season's worth of food in advance and pick up a weekly box of produce at the farm. Community Supported Agriculture supports small farms by providing income at the beginning of the season, when expenses are high and profits low, and by sharing the

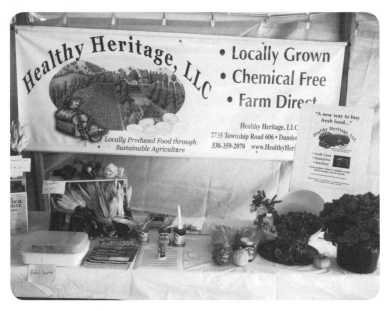

A CSA puts you in partnership with a farmer for the summer. Your advance payment helps the farmer plan their crops. You will then receive a weekly share of the harvest. Some farms will invite you to add "sweat equity" to your payment and join them in the fields for planting, weeding, or harvest.

risk of crop failures and the blessing of abundances. You can find CSA listings at www.localharvest.org and other websites, by word of mouth, or in the newspaper. The farmers' market is another good place to make CSA connections. Some CSAs require a few hours of labor from their members; others allow you to trade labor for a discounted rate. Some require you to pick up your weekly box of food at the farm, while others will deliver to a central meeting point in town.

Purchasing directly from farmers has its drawbacks, as Amy G. noted. "One disadvantage of local foods is that you can't get everything in one shopping trip. I usually end up driving to the farm once a week to pick up my food order, although we do share the burden with other families. But I realize that I have it easier than many people have, since I'm friends with the farmers and live only 15 minutes away."

If transportation is an obstacle, consider joining or forming a buying club. Find others who are also in search of local foods and save time and gas by taking turns driving to pick up items for the group. If you live in a large urban area, you may be able to find a farmer who already has a club set up in your area. Weston A. Price Foundation chapters can often help you make connections.

One farmer we met has organized several buying groups who purchase dairy, meat, produce, eggs, honey, and more. In one of the groups, about 20 families receive an e-mail listing what is available for the week and respond with their orders. Different people take turns making the one-hour trip to the farm to pick up orders and then take them to a distribution point.

Laura S. participated in another type of arrangement in Cleveland, called City Fresh. "City Fresh is a CSA-type arrangement organized by the New Agrarian Center; rather than being a commitment to only one farm, it's a collaboration of many. We participated for most of the summer and fall by purchasing a half share each week and picking it up at our local 'Fresh Stop' (luckily, only about a half mile from our house)."

If you want the convenience of home delivery, businesses like Wholesome Acres in northern Ohio and Door-to-Door Organics in several major cities offer a variety of online ordering services. As farmers and consumers collaborate, more of these options will likely become available, making local foods convenient even for urban buyers.

GROW YOUR OWN

You can't get any more local than your own backyard! We will cover gardening more extensively in chapter eight, but growing your own is an excellent way to provide yourself with fresh food throughout much of the year—even in small spaces. Gardening has benefits beyond just providing you with food; it is good for the environment, good for the community, and good for your health as well.

Neighbors and friends with gardens can also become local food sources, and finding ways to barter excess produce can be a good community builder. A garden may allow you to swap your surplus produce for things that you don't grow. For example, last summer Lisa was able to trade sweet corn for organic strawberries and cherries, and honey for maple syrup. Few of us can grow everything we need, but growing a little extra might allow you to swap for something you don't grow. You may look at your excess garden produce in a whole new way when you envision its bartering potential.

LACK OF AVAILABILITY

Even now, there are many areas even in the United States where people do not have reliable access to nutritious, reasonably priced foods, let alone locally grown ones. Termed "food deserts," these areas are increasingly common in both urban and rural locales. Many times these food deserts have developed as people have moved to the suburbs, and as big box stores have put smaller grocers out of business. For those without reliable transportation, the increasing distance makes healthy food less and less accessible.

One way to combat the food desert effect is to support small, local farms and shops—help keep them in business! Ramona N. is an urban nurse who is well aware of the challenges of finding fresh, local food in the city. "My favorite sources of local food are Sunny Slope orchard, an Amish farm where I buy eggs, Miller's blueberries, and

Vogley's fruit farm. The challenge is that each of these places is at least a half hour away. Sometimes I run out of items before I'm going that direction, or I stock up too much and things spoil.

"One obstacle to providing 'local' food to the city is that transportation is time/energy consuming. The food needs to sell before it spoils, yet suppliers need to either stock enough that people won't make a trip and find a small selection, or find a way to advertise what they do have. Most of my neighbors do not have Internet access in their homes."

A WAY OF LIFE

Critics of the "eat local" movement often charge that it is cheaper and more fuel-efficient to import things from climates where they grow easily than to eat the local version. To use an extreme example, if you live in Alaska, it's obviously going to take many resources to produce oranges there. It would take fewer resources to eat oranges from somewhere else, the critics argue. And they are correct—up to a point. However, they ignore the third and best option, which is to shift your diet to the kinds of foods that thrive in your own climate. In our Alaskan example, this would mean giving up the oranges and eating blueberries or some other kind of fruit that grows well in Alaska instead. By making such a shift, our hypothetical Alaskan could minimize the environmental impact of their meals while still supporting local farmers and businesses.

We asked Andrea G. how her family manages to eat locally. Her reply: "It is hard to answer, because it is just how we do it. The big 'mart'-type store is the last resort for something we need. If we see a roadside stand, we stop to look. We connect with friends who grow or raise something we do not, and try to work a trade for something that we have that they need. When we moved to a new town, I took advantage of my daily walks to look for neighbors who sold eggs from their backyard hens, extra garden produce, and such. I don't really think of even being 'intentional' as much as this is just the way of life for our family. We've built it into our children's thinking that this is the way to go—seek local first."

Finding local foods can seem overwhelming or impossible at first, but with practice, it will become part of your routine; a way of life. Most of us will probably need to rely on a combination of the strategies in this chapter to eat locally—for instance, a typical meal at the Amstutz house might consist of meat from a nearby farm, salad from our garden topped with a locally produced salad dressing from the grocery store, and Ohio potatoes from the farmers' market or grocery store. In summer and fall, a higher percentage of our food comes from roadside stands, farmers' markets, and our own garden; the rest of the year, we rely mostly on what we have in storage and the grocery store. The longer we eat this way, the less we even think about it. Treasure hunting for local foods has become our way of life.

Cindy S., a graphic designer, told us a story about her husband's transformation. "My husband is a big-city kid and I have deep roots in rural Ohio. We were newly married and were at the grocery store, talking about what we would like to eat. He wanted squash. I turned and went to the produce section and picked up some squash but noticed that he was not behind me. I searched for him and found him in the frozen foods section. He was holding a box. I said, 'What is that?' 'Squash,' he said. I never knew squash came in a box and he had no idea what was in the cart. Today, 34 years later, he makes the best squash dishes with no boxes involved!"

STEPS TO TAKE

1. Research what local food options exist in your region and learn the local brand names in your area. Visit one local business or farm this week.

2. Call or visit several markets to see what may fit into your regular shopping routine.

3. Encourage others to join you and consider organizing a buying club.

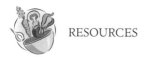

RESOURCES

1. *The Farmers' Market Book: Growing Food, Cultivating Community* by Jennifer Meta Robinson and J. A. Hartenfeld

2. *Sharing the Harvest: A Citizens Guide to Community Supported Agriculture, Revised and Expanded* by Elizabeth Henderson and Robyn Van En

A FREEZER FULL OF MEAT

Buying "freezer meat"—a whole, half, or quarter of an animal—is an economical way to get high-quality local meats but there are a few tricks to making the most of your purchase.

A quarter of beef or a side of hog, lamb, or goat may come with unfamiliar cuts like shanks, soup bones, cube steak, oxtail, organ meats, necks, or ham hocks. A 7-8-hour bake on low (or 3-4 hours on high) in a slow cooker is generally a safe way to try something new and make sure it comes out tender. Organ meats like heart and oxtail are delicious this way, as are roasts. For an easy one-dish meal, add quartered potatoes and slices of onion, carrot, and celery to the slow cooker along with your roast. The drippings and any leftover meat can be used the following day to make soup—just add vegetables, noodles or barley, and spices to taste.

If some cuts arrive in larger quantities than you normally use, perhaps you can stretch them into two or more meals. A round steak, for example, might be used in a stroganoff one night and the remainder broiled another night. You can also freeze extra portions of cooked meat and broth for "convenience" meals later.

For cuts with a lot of bone and small amount of meat in difficult crevices, like neck pieces or soup bones, cover with water and simmer for several hours with salt, pepper, onion, garlic, and herbs to create a delicious soup broth. Various steak cuts may be grilled but also make delicious stir-fries, kebabs, curries, etc.

Grass-fed ground meats such as hamburger and sausage often contain very little fat. This makes them an excellent value, since you aren't paying for fat that will be discarded, but you may want to add olive oil or some other fat when browning them. Another option is to simply add a little water to the pan to prevent the meat from sticking. Cooking times for cuts like steaks should be reduced by about 30% since the fat content is lower. When in doubt about cooking procedures, consult a good basic cookbook or ask the farmer directly, as they may have recipes and ideas to share.

Planning your menus a day or two ahead will give your meat time to thaw in the refrigerator, using less energy than quick-thawing methods. See Appendix A for more meat recipes.

TASTE OF SUMMER MEATBALLS

3# grass-fed hamburger	½ C. chopped onions
½ C. chopped peppers	2 cloves garlic, minced
2 eggs	1 C. quick oatmeal
¼ C. spaghetti sauce	2 T. Dijon mustard
¾ C. chopped tomatoes	2 T. fresh, chopped oregano
salt to taste	

Combine ingredients in a large bowl. Roll into 2" balls and bake at 350° for 45 minutes. - K.G.

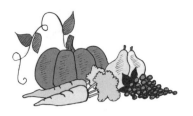

CHAPTER 5

Serving up the Harvest

I was 32 when I started cooking; up until then, I just ate.
- Julia Child

Now that you're finding new sources of local foods, the next step is to figure out how to prepare them. Some may be unfamiliar, like Patty Pan squash, bok choy, leeks, or tarragon. Making use of the foods you find at the farmers' market or in your CSA basket requires some knowledge of food preparation; otherwise they can too easily end up in the compost pile. Cooking skills are a vital link in learning to use the grand variety of fresh local foods in ways that your family will appreciate, and will bring many new flavors into your life.

A KITCHEN REVIVAL

In recent decades, cooking was reduced to a lowly task as people began to see prepared and canned foods as an efficient way to acquire nutrition so they could spend their valuable time on something more lucrative or entertaining than peeling potatoes or chopping onions. Nearly half of all U.S. food dollars are spent on restaurant or take-out food rather than on basics from the grocery store, and recent generations have not learned cooking skills from their parents and grandparents as they did in the past. However, the increasing popularity of the Food Network and several celebrity chefs is bringing food preparation back into fashion. One farmers' market vendor credits the Food Network with increasing business at her Saturday market as more folks learn cooking skills in the privacy of their home and want to experiment with fresh market items. Though some food celebrities could use a lesson in using healthy ingredients from local sources, this renewed interest in cooking may provide a boost to the local foods movement.

If prepared foods and convenience items currently consume your budget, learning to cook with basic fresh ingredients will quickly lower your food costs. *Animal, Vegetable, Miracle: A Year of Food Life* chronicles author Barbara Kingsolver's year of eating close to home. In this inspiring book she states, "Cooking is the great divide between good eating and bad. The gains are quantifiable: cooking and eating at home, even with quality ingredients, costs pennies on the dollar compared with meals prepared by a restaurant or factory."[30] Many of Kingsolver's stories describe how meal preparation and preserving food for the winter have become part of her family's culture—rituals that are done together and with great love. Perhaps if cooking together was marketed as a family bonding activity or a great entertainment alternative to watching a movie, it might become commonplace to see families sitting around together shelling peas, stuffing peppers, or peeling apples for pie.

> "*Food is fundamental to life, nourishing us in body and soul. The preparation of food strengthens our connection to nature. And the sharing of food immeasurably enriches our sense of community,*" is the first principle of the Chef's Collaborative.
> - *www.chefscollaborative.org*

Viewing food preparation as a valuable family activity might also lead to a revival of the practice of eating together around the table—a practice that is becoming a lost art in our fast-paced, convenience-driven culture. Studies show that children who eat dinner with their families have a healthier diet, do better in school, are less likely to experiment with drugs and alcohol, and feel better about themselves and their future.

---

30   Kingsolver, Barbara, Camille Kingsolver, and Steven L. Hopp, *Animal, Vegetable, Miracle: A Year of Food Life*. (HarperCollins: 2007) 129.

STARTING WITH PREMIUM INGREDIENTS

"Cooking is 80% ingredients," says chef Charlie Trotter of Charlie Trotter's Restaurant in Chicago. Years ago, chef training focused on cooking skills without a significant emphasis on ingredient sources. Today, most reputable culinary schools heavily stress the importance of starting with the best ingredients possible. However, you do not need to attend culinary school to achieve stellar results in the kitchen. Even the most novice cook can make a gourmet meal by starting with high-quality ingredients, purchased fresh locally. Flavor is an inherent trait in these fresh foods, not something that needs to be added with sauces, seasonings, and the like. A freshly picked salad that you toss together will taste better than any elaborate version made from pre-bagged lettuce simply because the lettuce is so much fresher and often includes varieties that never appear on supermarket shelves.

Chef Mike Mariola, owner of the South Market Bistro in Wooster, OH, agrees. "When I started cooking in restaurants that used sustainable products, I was encouraged to do that because the quality was so much better with the organic products. As a chef, if you're passionate about cooking and you have a hydroponic tomato vs. a vine-ripened tomato that's grown locally in season, it makes such a world of difference. Part of my motivation in using these products is that they're so much better."

Small-scale farmers who sell their products locally often pay careful attention to the details that give their products premium flavor. They choose the tastiest varieties, work to keep their soil and animals healthy, and handle their products with care; these are food artisans who are passionate about their product. Factory farms, by contrast, tend to focus on high yields, transportability, and the bottom line. In some cases, the owners may never even set foot on the ground they own. It's no surprise that artisan foods just taste better.

Some of these artisan foods can capture top dollar—goat cheeses, wines, specialty sauces—and their price tags reflect the intensive labor that goes into producing such high-quality products. However, if items like this don't fit your budget, the good news is that you can still eat like a gourmet without pinching your pocketbook. As the famous gastronome Curnonsky said, "Cuisine is when food tastes like it's supposed to." Start by substituting basic local, seasonal foods in your cooking, and you will begin to taste a difference. Simple food can be gourmet when the ingredients are good, and good ingredients can stand alone, without a lot of condiments or exotic additions.

Take tomatoes, for example. When you carry in a handful of soft, ripe tomatoes from your backyard or farmers' market, you can smell the flavor even before you slice them. It's hard to resist eating homegrown tomatoes on the spot. Our children often wander through the garden, eating them whole. If you want to go gourmet, just sprinkle a little olive oil and fresh basil on top. Out-of-season tomatoes, on the other hand, aren't good for much besides softball practice or maybe adding extra volume to a burger, doused with plenty of ketchup.

Biting into the dripping sweetness of a vine-ripened tomato is not a pleasure reserved for the rich and famous. It is accessible to anyone who can tuck a tomato plant into their flowerbed or take the time to find fresh tomatoes at a farmers' market or roadside stand.

Freshness and variety make a huge difference in salads as well. Once you try a salad of fresh mixed greens like romaine, kale, arugula, and endive, there is no going back to the limp, precut salads you once settled for. A good salad doesn't need much in the way of toppings or dressings to look and taste fabulous—just let the quality of the ingredients shine through. Greens are also easy to grow—even indoors! A few pots in the windowsill can keep you in fresh greens year-round.

Once you have purchased premium fresh ingredients close to home, a first step in using them effectively is properly cleaning and storing your produce. Proper storage temperature and technique will help fruits and vegetables maintain optimum freshness until you are ready to use them. Some things are best used immediately, like fragile heirloom tomatoes that are known for their flavor, not their shelf life, or just-picked sweet corn whose sugars rapidly turn to starch as time passes. Fresh herbs keep best in the fridge in a glass of water like a flower bouquet, except for basil, which prefers warmer temperatures. Other produce, such as properly washed and stored greens, can keep well for several days in a crisper drawer while sturdy crops like cabbage and beets will last even longer. Potatoes, onions, and garlic will keep for weeks, even months, when stored in a cool, dark place. See Appendix B for a produce storage chart.

LEARNING NEW SKILLS

Deb G., a college university chef during the school year and a market gardener in the summer months, sees teaching cooking skills as vital to her farming success. As people gain cooking knowledge, demand for her produce increases. Deb observes that many people

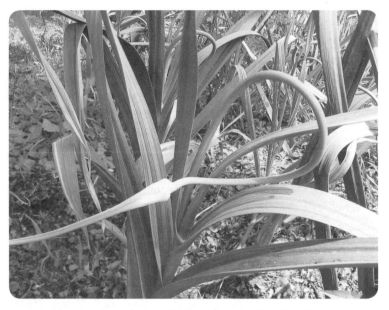

Many recipes are enhanced by the pungency of garlic, which is easily grown in most regions of the United States and readily available at farmers' markets. This garlic plant just sent out a flower scape. The scape can be cut and used to add mild garlic flavor to salads or stir-fries before the bulb is ready to harvest.

perceive cooking as too hard or feel intimidated by recipes with too many ingredients, and sometimes the convenience of buying things already prepared is just too tempting. So she teaches various cooking classes that focus on using seasonal produce and encourage people to try new recipes.

One of Deb's favorite tips for beginners is to learn to make vinaigrettes (using natural sweeteners) to use on salads, stir-fried veggies, and marinated meats. She combines ingredients like olive oil, fresh herbs, garlic, lemon juice, honey, salt, and pepper and keeps some vinaigrette on hand for making these quick dishes. When using herbs, Deb suggests starting with the most familiar like parsley and basil and working your way up to more exotic ones. Like many things in life, cooking is a skill best learned in steps, with the most important step being getting started. Don't give up if your first attempts do not turn out well!

HONEY LIME VINAIGRETTE (DEB GEISER)

Yield: 1 cup

$^{1}/_{3}$ C. vegetable oil	¼ C. rice vinegar
¼ C. honey	2 T. spicy mustard
1 T. cilantro, chopped	1 lime, juiced
1 tsp. sesame oil	1 T. red pepper, minced
1 T. red onion, minced	salt and pepper to taste

Combine vegetable oil, rice vinegar, honey, mustard, lime juice, and sesame oil in a small saucepan. Heat over medium-high heat for 1-2 minutes, or until the mixture begins to bubble. Remove from heat and continue to whisk for 1 minute—this emulsifies the dressing and it should thicken as it cools. Add the minced vegetables and cilantro, season to taste with salt and pepper. Cover, let set for two hours before serving.

-For more vinaigrette recipes from Deb, see Appendix A.

There are many excellent cookbooks on the market, including several recent books focused specifically on seasonal produce from the farmers' market (see resources). The benefit of these cookbooks is that they pair items found in the same season, like strawberries and rhubarb or tomatoes and zucchini, to create combination dishes that do not require purchasing produce from far away. Additionally, most call for fresh herbs rather than excess salt, ketchup, or mayonnaise as flavor enhancers.

Sometimes a CSA will offer a weekly newsletter including recipes, or farmers' market stands will provide recipe ideas for the produce they are selling. You might also ask the farmer or other shoppers how they prepare the veggies they are selecting. Most cooks are glad to share information about their family favorites. I (Karen) enjoy encouraging customers to try out the herbs that come with their weekly veggie baskets. One grandmotherly customer was quite hesitant at first in trying unfamiliar things, but after specific suggestions about which herbs to pair with beans or potatoes she was convinced. Soon she started requesting her favorites: lemon basil and rosemary. This year she even planted lemon basil and rosemary in her flowerbed so she can have access to them anytime she wants. It's never too late to learn and enjoy new pleasures in life!

EQUIPPING YOUR KITCHEN

A few basic tools are necessary to cook from scratch. Cookbooks with color pictures, that emphasize basic cooking skills, are a good place to start. A cooking pot, skillet, knives, and a cutting board are all you really need to begin. However, quality tools certainly do make cooking more pleasant. Home parties selling quality kitchen tools are quite popular. (Unfortunately, their utensils are usually demonstrated with semi-processed foods and out-of-season produce.) If your goal is to include more produce, pass on the potato chip canisters and fancy can openers and invest in good knives and solid cookware instead. These items are available at department stores, specialty cooking shops, online stores, Lehman's, and many other places. If you are on a tight budget, check garage sales and thrift stores first to find bargains.

I've had to update and upgrade some of my kitchen equipment. I remember someone once said her most important kitchen utensil was a scissors to open the bags of salad. For years, I had an electric can opener on the countertop—no more. Now on the rare occasion I need one, I use a handheld one. However, I've had to invest in various tools such as sharp knives, cutting boards, large stockpots, and canning equipment. I like the idea that glass canning jars and plastic freezer boxes can be reused year after year rather than throwing out packaging or trusting the waste management people to recycle cans and cardboard. This winter I finally got one of those "professional" electric mixers with a dough hook, slicer, shredder, and grinding attachment. The Amish have similar low-tech versions of these, which they consider a necessity—along with their expensive stainless steel cookware and cutlery. A pot of soup and home-baked bread is a great way to stay warm (and at home) in the winter. Out of bread? Bake some.

-*Joanne L.*

Taking the time to use these basic tools can become a stress reliever—a time to meditate or think about those for whom you are preparing the food. Food processors speed up the job of chopping veggies significantly, but the Slow Food movement also emphasizes the value of learning to do these acts by hand and enjoying the process of food preparation. Meal preparation and clean-up times can also become a special time to talk with a spouse, child, or friend.

TIME-CRUNCH COOKING

Cooking does require time and planning, but there are many ways to fit it into a busy lifestyle. In the Geiser household, the simplest way to put food on the table on a busy day is to serve it in its natural state—a basket of fresh berries, a bowl of unshelled peas or a plate of cherry tomatoes, cucumber slices, and broccoli florets. During the summer season, we take a basket out to the garden and gather what is ripe. Then we brainstorm a meal using the gathered ingredients which often is a stir-fry (see Appendix A for our favorite combos) or veggies mixed with rice or pasta.

When time is short, good planning can help you put quick, healthy meals on the table with a minimum of effort. Making a double batch of soup and freezing some, creating a weekly menu using seasonal items, and keeping a good supply of staples on hand will all save precious minutes and allow for home-cooked convenience. Using a slow cooker is another way to provide home-cooked meals even in a time crunch. See chapter seven for more tips on making local foods more convenient.

THE ART OF HOSPITALITY

These days, inviting people over for a home-cooked meal is a rare occurrence. It's much easier to go out to eat together or simply order pizza. Some families, however, are attempting to bring old-fashioned hospitality back into their lives, using local foods as a foundation.

Angie B. and her husband and young daughters enjoy sharing good food with guests in their small country home. Rather than being taken to a restaurant, out-of-town family and friends are treated to a home-cooked meal based on local foods. Meats from a local farm become delicious grilled chicken, roasted rosemary chicken, or sloppy joes. Fresh veggies from their garden round out the menu, along

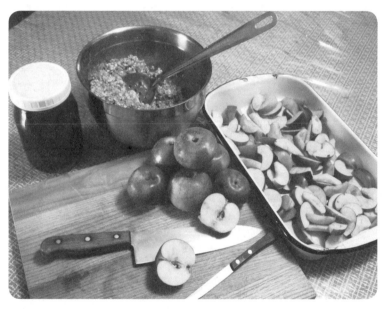

Incorporating local foods into your diet will require a basic supply of kitchen equipment. You may also need to spend more time in your kitchen. The extra efforts will be worth it as your family enjoys the many benefits of eating closer to home.

with apples or peaches from a nearby orchard in a pie or cobbler for dessert. "We are a good team; my husband likes to grill and I love to bake (especially using our outdoor Dutch oven), so being able to share the results of that partnership with others is very rewarding," says Angie. "It is valuable to us to be able to serve our guests truly good food and it has become an excellent way to educate them on the virtues of locally grown food—they do notice a difference."

ANGIE'S DUTCH OVEN APPLE COBBLER

Filling:
8 C. thinly sliced apples (we like Cortland or McIntosh)
2 tsp. cinnamon
1 C. sugar
½ tsp. nutmeg

Place apples in buttered Dutch oven. In a small bowl, combine sugar and spices. Sprinkle and stir into apples.

Topping:

1½ C. unbleached flour	½ tsp. salt
½ C. whole-wheat flour	2 eggs, beaten
1 C. sugar	1 C. milk
2 tsp. baking powder	½ C. butter, melted

In a large mixing bowl, combine dry ingredients. In a small bowl, mix the wet ingredients, then pour into dry ingredients and mix until smooth. Pour the batter over the apples. Bake at 350° for 45 min. or until golden brown in an oven or fire pit.

Another family has kept the spirit of hospitality alive in their home and I (Karen) frequently get calls asking if I have extra salad available for their weekend guests. Jill B. and her family regularly host family, out-of-town guests, and even college presidents and church leaders. Jill writes, "Serving guests in our home is one way we try to say 'Welcome' to them in a deeper and more intimate way than we could by taking them to a restaurant. We share our home, our family, and our food (purchased locally as much as possible) which is intentionally prepared with lots of care. It is definitely time consuming to prepare for guests but is very fulfilling for our whole family.

"I always look forward to getting my salad bag assortments from Karen. The greens are so fresh and delicious, and the colorful edible flowers add beauty and just the right amount of whimsy to our dinner table. The salads garner plenty of 'oohs' and 'aahs' because of their lovely presentation but are equally enjoyed because of their wonderful freshness, taste, and variety of textures."

Inviting others over for a meal doesn't need to be an elaborate, overwhelming affair. Try out meals on your family ahead of time and choose recipes that can be prepared in advance for your first attempts at cooking for others and whenever you are on a tight schedule. Consider asking your guests to bring a dish that fits a simple theme, such as soup and bread, or curry with toppings. Elaborate meals and fancy place settings are not requirements for being a good host. A hearty welcome, thoughtfully prepared food, and lively table conversation will bless the guests who enter your home with the gift of hospitality.

CONCLUSION

If cooking isn't a skill you grew up with, don't despair! Local foods, a few basic tools, and many excellent resources can give you a fast start. If you are already a gourmet, incorporating fresh, local foods will open new horizons of flavor. No matter what your level of kitchen expertise, adding to your repertoire of cooking skills will save money, benefit your family's health, and introduce new pleasures. Sharing that good food through hospitality will extend those benefits far beyond your own household.

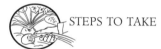 STEPS TO TAKE

1. Buy a good seasonal cookbook, such as *Simply in Season*, to learn how to cook unfamiliar foods. Other good titles include *The Farmers' Market Cookbook* by Richard Ruben, *Local Flavors* by Deborah Madison, and *Saving Dinner* by Leanne Ely. Try a new recipe using foods that are in season in your area.

2. Gather as a family to eat around the table one more time per week than you currently do.

3. Look for opportunities to learn cooking skills—The Food Network, cooking classes, helping Grandma, etc.

4. Help revive the art of hospitality by inviting someone over for a meal using local foods.

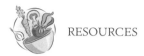

RESOURCES

1. *The Victory Garden Cookbook* by Marian Morash

2. *Farmer John's Cookbook: The Real Dirt on Vegetables* by Farmer John Peterson

3. *The Surprising Power of Family Meals* by Miriam Weinstein

4. *Animal, Vegetable, Miracle* by Barbara Kingsolver with Steven Hopp and Camille Kingsolver

SAVORING THE SEASONS: INSPIRATIONS FROM A CHEF

For those of us who are gardeners, spring and summer's garden bounty is bliss! When a crop arrives in great profusion, we often focus on recipes that showcase that one item, but we can increase our enjoyment by combining it with other seasonal foods. Toss out monoculture and take a more global approach to creatively combining the many choices available in the garden, whether it's early spring, the full bloom of summer, or fall harvest.

Sometimes we're eager to enjoy the latest arrivals but find there's really not quite enough yet to harvest to make a substantial contribution to any given meal. I've compiled some ideas for food combining that will add interest and help you enjoy the first envoys along with the harvest that's in full swing or maybe even on its way out.

In the spring, I look forward to asparagus but find that early on I have just a few spears to work with. To preview their long-awaited arrival, I combine them with a few baby carrots, some snow peas, and all the spinach I can spare. Steamed and tossed with Beurre Blanc or creamery butter, fresh tarragon, and chervil or parsley, the result is colorful and fabulous.

SPRING MEDLEY

Beurre Blanc:

¼ C. dry white wine
2 T. finely chopped shallot
¼ C. white wine vinegar
6-8 T. cold butter, cut into small pieces
½ pound fresh asparagus, cleaned and cut into 3" lengths
8 slender carrots, halved lengthwise
½ pound of edible-pod and/or snow peas
1 slender leek, washed and cut into 2" lengths, then cut
    into ¼" strips (you may substitute 4 slender green onions)
a profusion of fresh spinach or Swiss chard removed from
    the stems and cut into ¼" strips
small amounts of chervil, tarragon and parsley

Begin by preparing the Beurre Blanc and/or chopping the herbs of your choice. For the Beurre Blanc, put the vinegar, wine, and shallot and a pinch of salt in a saucepan and cook until reduced in half. Turn off the heat and whisk in the butter piece by piece until it is well blended. It should be thick and white. Set aside.

Next, steam the carrots and asparagus for 3-4 minutes; add the peas and steam for another 3 minutes. Then add the spinach and/or Swiss chard and steam until just wilted. Transfer to a serving bowl and toss immediately with the butter and minced fresh herbs or toss with 2-3 T. of Beurre Blanc. Serve immediately.

I love beans. Green, yellow, purple, Roma, slender, foot long, flat. I do several plantings so I can extend the season as long as possible. Here are a few ideas for serving beans throughout the season. Prepared simply or exotically, I love beans!

One of my favorite things to do is to combine different types, like yellow, green, and Roma beans. I steam them separately to accommodate their cooking times so I end up with crisp, tender beans. In this case, I usually toss the Romas into the steamer first and give them a two-minute head start before adding the yellow beans and greens. I also pay attention to size to determine when the others should be added to the pot. As a rule, if you enjoy crisp, tender beans, steam them for 8-10 minutes. I enjoy them simply tossed with butter or olive oil and seasoned with salt and pepper.

Try seasoning beans with fresh summer savory or fresh marjoram. A tablespoon of fresh herbs should suffice. Often I'll toss two generous handfuls of Swiss chard (free from stems and cut into ¼" strips) into the pot for the last minute of cooking, just enough to wilt them and preserve their rich nutrients. Combining yellow wax beans with Swiss chard makes a lovely presentation.

GREEN BEANS TOSSED WITH ROASTED GARLIC & ARUGULA

4 C. packed fresh arugula	1 bulb garlic
1 lb. green beans, cleaned and trimmed	¼ C. olive oil

To roast the garlic, peel and trim each clove and place in a small ramekin. Cover with olive oil, making sure the oil completely covers them. Cover tightly with a lid or a double thickness of aluminum foil. Bake in preheated 375° oven for 20-30 minutes or until garlic cloves are tender and light golden brown. Check after 20 minutes. When the garlic is ready, remove with a slotted spoon and set aside; reserve the oil.

Place the beans in a large steamer and steam for 8-10 minutes or until crisp tender. Add the arugula and steam just long enough to wilt. Transfer the beans and arugula to a serving bowl. Toss with garlic cloves, some of the reserved olive oil, and salt and pepper to taste.

-Monique Theoret is a chef/caterer who enjoys using local, sustainably grown and seasonal ingredients in her cooking.

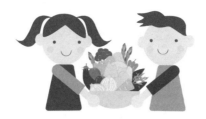

CHAPTER 6

Bringing the Children on Board

The day is coming when children will start telling their grandparents to eat their spinach.
- Charles Benbrook

As an adult, you might enjoy eggplant parmesan with a side salad of arugula and endive—but what about the children? What if French fries and ketchup are the only vegetables they'll touch, or they only eat chicken disguised as nuggets? Getting the younger generation hooked on fresh, local foods can be challenging, but it is a change that can transform both their health and their future world.

CHILDHOOD OBESITY

Considering the epidemic of childhood obesity in the United States, it is more important than ever to educate our children on the importance of wise food choices. Daily bombardment with commercials for processed foods, flashy supermarket displays, and the allure of sugary snacks can be hard for young consumers to resist. Marketing for dead, processed foods is overwhelming, and parents need to counter that with their own "marketing" of the fresh, local fruits, veggies, dairy, and meats that should be the foundation of a child's diet.

Dr. Susan Okie, in her eye-opening book *Fed Up! Winning the War Against Childhood Obesity* observes, "Most parents are eager to take action when told their child is sick. It's much more difficult to persuade families to make major alterations in their lifestyle when children seem to be well, merely to prevent disease sometime in the future. Yet that's what we must do. When doctors and public health officials tell us that almost one-third of our children are sick with obesity or are at risk of becoming so, it's time for us to change our children's environment, both inside and outside the home, in ways that will help them build leaner and healthier bodies."[31] The family dinner table and local foods full of freshness and nutrition can be crucial weapons in the battle against childhood obesity.

PERSUADE THEM WITH FLAVOR

A large part of the battle is getting children to taste-test fully ripe, in-season produce after they have been turned off by the lack of flavor of out-of-season, industrial varieties. They may be convinced that all peas are tasteless or that greens are always limp and

> "*My favorite vegetables are Brussels sprouts, red beets, sweet corn, and lima beans. But I'll pass on the spinach and weird things like bok choy." -Reuben, age 12*

bitter. Or perhaps the only green beans or corn they know is the canned version, with much of the flavor cooked out. Once they've tried fresh young vegetables, most children can't resist the taste. Local foods offer a wonderful opportunity to introduce your children to the full sweetness and flavor of fresh produce.

Our children's birthday menu choices are often quite revealing. In the Geiser household, red beets are a frequent choice along with salads (made with Buttercrunch lettuce, hold the weird greens), roasted chicken with rosemary, mashed potatoes or baked fat fries, and sugar snap peas. Children often surprise us. Heidi S., age 5, loved the yellow Persimmon tomatoes she sampled at a fall Harvest Festival. Her mom reports, "Heidi said, 'It's so good, I can't stop eating it!' She kept wanting to eat more before we left. I had never thought to try yellow tomatoes and was surprised that she did. We plan to add a plant or two of Persimmons to our small garden at home next year." Encourage your children to be adventurous and try new tastes—they might just like them!

---

31   Susan Okie, *Fed Up! Winning the War Against Childhood Obesity* (Joseph Henry Press: 2006) 23.

STARTING YOUNG

Starting with good food at a young age is ideal. Establishing a palate that is accustomed to food in its natural state lays a good foundation for later years. Many baby foods are laden with additives, so preparing your own first foods from organic, whole fruits, vegetables, and grains is a great alternative. Baby foods are simple

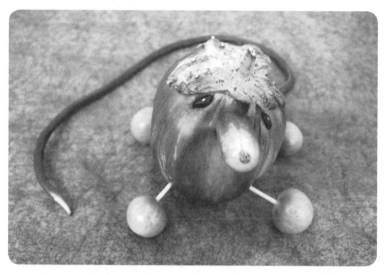

When started young, children quickly develop a taste for fresh vegetables. Getting them into the habit of eating cherry tomatoes, fresh carrots and cucumber slices rather than processed foods will benefit them for life. One way to get children more excited about eating vegetables is to hand them a few toothpicks and let them create veggie art.

to make; simply puree cooked vegetables such as squash, carrots, or peas and freeze them into ice cube trays to create easy-to-use, single servings. Certainly, high-quality baby food brands do exist, but learning to make your own from the best local ingredients is an economical alternative and gets the family in practice for future cooking with fresh ingredients.

Corrie Y., mother of two young children, reports, "Many of our daughter's first solid foods were from our garden or a local organic farm; things like butternut squash, sweet potatoes, and fruit. As a toddler, she would roam through our garden eating peas, cherry tomatoes, greens, and broccoli. Even though she is little, we try to explain why these foods are healthy and good for her. We hope that by introducing good food early she will be able to make healthy choices throughout life."

For those who haven't had the benefit of that good start, there is still hope for changing what your children eat. As you gradually add fresh, local foods to your family's diet, their taste buds will gravitate to the more flavorful and healthy options. Replacing empty junk food calories with less-processed, nutrient-dense food is a major step toward helping our children stay at a healthy weight.

COOKING FOODS THEY WILL EAT

Some fresh foods will definitely be new and need to be introduced gradually and pleasingly. Fresh sugar snap peas or cherry tomatoes may be a better first-time choice than bok choy or leeks. A pile of unfamiliar green stuff on a supper plate can be an instant turnoff to children. Start with recipes that your family already likes and add in some locally grown ingredients. For example, add small green bean chunks to a favorite casserole or finely shredded spinach or greens to soup rather than serving those vegetables on their own.

Another option is to look at the processed foods your children regularly eat and brainstorm a replacement. If you find a good source of grain, try oatmeal topped with berries, or serve blueberry muffins instead of cereal out

"*My favorite way to eat lettuce is to hold a Buttercrunch lettuce heart, put a radish in the center, add a dollop of Ranch dressing, and eat it like an ice-cream cone.*" -Elizabeth, age 9

of a box. Popsicles made from yogurt, fruit in season (strawberries, peaches, raspberries, blueberries, even pumpkin), and a bit of honey whirled in the blender are enjoyable on a hot day. Delicious fat potato fries are easy to bake in your oven and if your children enjoy novelty, you might even try mashed potatoes using blue potatoes if they are available. Shredded zucchini can be effectively hidden in a number of baked goods including brownies, and some moms have even been known to sneak shredded yellow squash into macaroni and cheese. If you're desperate and need more tips on sneaking vegetables into your children's meals, see the resources at the end of this chapter for two cookbooks that elaborate on this technique.

As you try new recipes on your family, take careful notes on what worked and what flopped. Don't give up too quickly when some dishes aren't fully appreciated. It may take eight or ten exposures before a child is willing to accept a new food. Continue experimenting in small batches and work at instilling an adventurous attitude toward food. "I get a lot of eye-rolling from my teenagers when I present new foods at the table from the garden or our CSA basket," says Kelly S. "Fortunately, it's all in jest because they usually end up liking what I serve. Everyone's used to me trying new vegetables and herbs, and they laugh at my 'new recipes' but tell me later they are appreciative. I wouldn't miss the eye-rolls for the world!"

Experimenting with fresh herbs in cooking is a good way to get children excited about trying new things. Rosemary with chicken and potatoes, basil on tomatoes, chives snipped on baked potatoes, and fresh dill on pickles are good starters. Adding new flavors in small amounts is key, because overdoing some stronger herbs like lovage or sage can turn children off in a hurry.

A bonus with fresh produce is that not all of it needs to be cooked and many things taste best raw. Cucumber slices, cherry tomatoes, and sugar snap peas make great snacks for nibbling. Or try washing carrots with the greens still on for children to eat like rabbits. Melons and fruits need only be sliced. If you're feeling extra creative, you can even make "food creatures," like peppers with cherry tomato eyes, baby zucchini boats, or blueberry snowmen. Joost Elffers has written a whole series of books featuring a host of adorable food creatures— your public library probably carries some.

If your children are still hesitant to try new dishes, another trick is to include them in the cooking process. When children make their own culinary creations, they are more likely to try a taste and find they like it. Teaching them the age-appropriate skills of measuring, cutting, following recipes, and safe stove usage will benefit them many times over in the future. There are many good children's cookbooks available to get you started, or you can simply use basic recipes that you enjoy. Give them an apron and a few kitchen tools and spend a fun afternoon cooking together.

If none of these tips works for your children, we have one last sure-fire recommendation: put ketchup on it!

TAKING THEM TO THE SOURCE

It can be amusing when children believe that their milk originates at the store and that a "real" carrot is a uniformly chiseled orange stub rather than a bundle of long, tapered ones still sporting their green tops. Such confusion is not limited to children, as we recently saw a potato chip ad that pictured workers plucking potatoes off bushes with no shovels in sight, when in reality potatoes grow underground. Such misinformation is a sad commentary on how far we have strayed from our agricultural roots. In his book, *Last Child in the Woods: Saving our children from nature deficit disorder*, Richard Louv laments the loss of connection to our food sources. "In less than half a century, the culture has moved from a time when small family farms dominated the countryside to a transitional time when many suburban families' vegetable gardens provided little more than recreation, to the current age of shrink-wrapped, lab-produced food. In one way, young people are more aware of the sources of what they eat, such as conditions in confinement farming, which has moved many young people to vegetarianism. Such knowledge, however, does not necessarily mean that the young are personally involved with their food sources."[32] Eating local foods provides a valuable opportunity to reconnect both children and adults to the true roots of what we eat and can give a dietary education that goes far beyond any book or television documentary.

"*My favorite veggies are carrots. I also like eating raspberries with my grandpa in his berry patch.*" -Sean, age 4

A family visit to a pick-your-own berry patch is an opportunity to teach children about the source of their food and create some memories in the process. Take the children along if you are buying items directly from a farm or farmers' market and encourage them to ask the farmer questions about the animals, trees, or plants that

32   Louv, Richard. *Last Child in the Woods: Saving our children from nature deficit disorder* (Algonquin Books: 2008) 21.

produce the food you are purchasing. If you are part of a CSA that hosts workdays, let your children experience weeding and harvesting on the plot of ground their summer meals are coming from. When children have the opportunity to dig their own potatoes, pluck cherry tomatoes right from the vine, or gather fresh eggs, the taste is incomparable because there was effort and personal connection involved. This direct involvement has even been known to convince picky eaters to add something to their "favorite" list.

This spring I learned that a neighbor had an overabundance of asparagus. My 8-year-old daughter, Emma, went with me to pick up a bagful they had gladly reserved for us. I remembered my grandma's asparagus patch from when I was young so I asked my neighbor if we could see his garden. He told us that his mother had planted that asparagus patch back in the 1960s. After petting a few kittens and identifying a few flowers in the flowerbeds, we headed home.

We had roasted asparagus and garlic with supper that night. Emma, always willing to try a new food, had tried asparagus before and decided it wasn't on her list of favorite foods. She tried it again that night and declared it was much better than the previous time. (I used the same recipe!) Since then, every time we pass the neighbor's house, she says, "That's where we got the asparagus. Yum!" I like to think that someday asparagus will be on her list of favorite foods, along with other garden goodies, because of experiences like this one.

-Lisa Z. manages a World Crafts (fair trade) store. She is the mother of two pre-teens and is active in her church and community.

An outing to a farmers' market is an excellent way to expose children to the varieties and colors of ripe produce available. Let them smell, feel, and make some selections of their own. Some vendors may have samples or special freebies for children. Additionally, larger farm markets may run special events for children with petting zoos, a chance to dig for worms, or other educational activities.

"I liked helping my aunt grow and pick pumpkins. Once I even saw a butterfly come out of its cocoon in her garden." -Cole, age 8

Even supermarket shopping can be a teaching tool to help children learn to make good choices. Let them be detectives in finding out where food comes from. Teach them to read labels and learn as a family what foods come in each season. Show them the math by comparing the price of ready-made food versus a similar item made from scratch. When a tempting display of strawberries appears mid-winter, take the opportunity to share about why you wait for them to be in season in your locality.

GARDENING WITH CHILDREN

Including children in gardening is another excellent way to teach them about where their food comes from. Participating in the process of planting a seed in the earth and eating the results several months later is a good lesson in working towards a goal and literally enjoying the fruit of one's labor. Helping in the garden also doubles as an effective tactic to entice picky eaters to sample fresh vegetables.

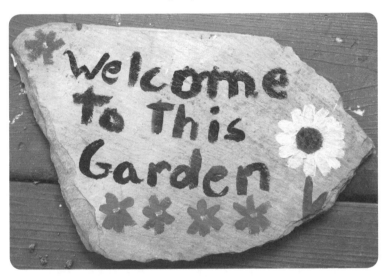

Even youngsters can get involved in the garden. Gardens are a great place to learn about natural systems, hard work and good food. They inspire creativity on many levels. A ten-year-old created this sign for her personal garden space.

Simple crops like radishes, potatoes, and beans are good ones to start with, and a single cherry tomato plant can provide bountiful returns for a youngster. If you want to be creative, child-friendly gardening can include bean teepees, sunflower houses, pizza gardens, and other unique themes.

The Geiser children each get a small plot of their own where they choose what to plant, care for it, and then eat the rewards. Cherry tomatoes and freshly pulled carrots are the "candy" of their gardens. Our preschool boys get a thrill out of planting a few hills of potatoes in their gardens, digging the buried treasure, and eating their own potatoes for supper. Each winter the children peruse the seed catalogs while I am making my selections for the year and add a few things to the list. This year my oldest son plans to raise four different colors of watermelons and my daughter wants to grow a pumpkin patch along with heirloom tomatoes.

Even if you don't have the time or space for your own garden, letting your children help a neighbor or grandparent can build a meaningful connection, both with the food they grow and with the gardener.

My father has a large garden and loves to share his bounty. We use squash, green beans, lettuce, tomatoes, onions, potatoes, soybeans, and asparagus from Dad. We can also pick blueberries, wild blackberries, and rhubarb if we like and make grape juice from Dad's Concord grapes. I like that our three children learn to try a variety of veggies and see Grandpa enjoy being in the garden even though it is a lot of hard work. He is a wonderful example to them. When we visit their grandmother in Michigan, she also likes to show off her garden to the children. She shares her bounty with us when we visit and we still have some turnips and acorn squash she sent home with us.

> "*I* like every vegetable that we grow in the garden. Just not the bizarre ones." -Katelyn, age 11

It seems like a small difference, but a small difference can make a big difference in your family, as we are called to care for and train our children to mature and run homes of their own some day. We are teaching them our habits, likes, and dislikes and they are watching. I believe the way we can most influence the world is through our children. They are watching everything we do and they model it. This can affect the choices they make, including their food choices.

- Kathy G. is a mother of three who plans to expand their small backyard garden and mini orchard to keep up with her family's growing appetites. She enjoys taking her children for "work bees" at relatives' gardens to both help and learn.

STORIES FROM THE CLASSROOM

Thanks to the vision of California chef Alice Waters, the Martin Luther King Jr. Middle School in Berkeley, California, added gardens to their curriculum and the resulting fresh produce to their cafeteria fare. Planning, planting, weeding, harvesting, and cooking are all part of the hands-on learning that these schoolchildren

"I like carrots, vegetables, beans, carrots, vegetables, and celery. And I don't like onions. I like flowers to smell and I like to eat buns. I like my flower in my garden." -Hannah, age 3

participate in. In the process, the children learn lessons on worms, ecology, food preparation, and even table manners. Alice writes, "The family meal has undergone a steady devaluation from its one-time role at the center of human life, when it was the daily enactment of shared necessity and ritualized cooperation. Today, as never before in history, the meals of children are likely to have been cooked by strangers, to consist of highly processed foods that are produced far away, and are likely to be taken casually, greedily, in haste, and, all too often, alone."[33] The Edible Schoolyard is a model program that offers resources for other schools, whether urban or rural, to include gardening into their school program.

It doesn't take a formal program to bring local foods to the classroom; some teachers are sharing their passions for good food by literally growing it in the classroom and taking other opportunities to share about food sources. Tony G. is a fourth-grade teacher in an inner-city school who finds many ways to incorporate healthy food training into the school day. He often takes produce purchased at the

---

33   www.edibleschoolyard.com

farmers' market to show the students and in the classroom is growing several herbs and a stevia plant. He also has shown the video *Super Size Me*, illustrating the ills of fast food along with the importance of reading food labels and making good choices in the cafeteria, and providing many other thought-provoking lessons about nutrition and local foods.

CONCLUSION

When you move from coaxing your children to try new fresh foods to watching them convince cautious young friends to try the fresh peaches or cherry tomatoes you just brought home from the farmers' market, you have made great strides toward a healthier future for your children. This accomplishment will benefit their health, childhood obesity rates, and future generations beyond measure. Indeed, it may someday be the children who encourage their grandparents to eat their spinach.

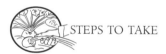 STEPS TO TAKE

1. Take your children along to the farmers' market or roadside stand and let them choose some veggies to add to your purchase.

2. Introduce a new vegetable or fruit to a family meal.

3. Let your children experience growing their own vegetables—in your backyard or by helping a grandparent or neighbor.

4. Consider helping to start an Edible Schoolyard program at a school in your community.

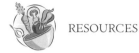

RESOURCES

1. *Blue Potatoes, Orange Tomatoes* by Rosalind Creasy

2. *Roots, Shoots, Buckets and Boots* by Sharon Lovejoy – creative ideas for children's gardening

3. *How Groundhog's Garden Grew* by Lynne Cherry

4. *Simply in Season Kid's Cookbook* by Mark Beach and Julie Kauffman

5. *The Sneaky Chef: Simple Strategies for Hiding Healthy Foods in Kid's Favorite Meals* by Missy Chase Lapine

6. *Deceptively Delicious* by Jessica Seinfeld

7. *The Omnivore's Dilemma for Kids: The Secrets Behind What You Eat* by Michael Pollan

YOGURT FRUIT SMOOTHIES OR POPSICLES

Add to blender: 3 C. yogurt, 1 C. fruit in season (strawberries, peaches, blueberries, raspberries, etc.), honey or other sweetener to taste, ½ tsp. vanilla.

Blend until smooth and enjoy as smoothies or pour into Popsicle molds and freeze for a delicious and nutritious summertime treat.

Here's a fresh, child-friendly summer/fall day's menu using some of the recipes in Appendix A. These recipes are not only fun for children to make but healthy and seasonal as well.

BREAKFAST	LUNCH	DINNER
Smoothies	Pita pizzas	Shish kebabs
Mini muffins	Fresh veggies, cut up	Potato wedges
Homemade butter		Garden salad
		Lemonade or mint tea

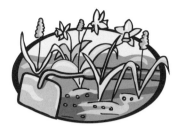

CHAPTER 7

Cost and Convenience

C ost and convenience are two of the biggest barriers to eating local for many families. At first glance, the price of some local foods may cause sticker shock, and with our busy lives, it seems there is just no extra time to shop or cook anymore. Nevertheless, many locavores find ways to overcome these obstacles. In this chapter, we will share tips from a variety of people who have discovered ways to make local foods both affordable and convenient.

Busy people may be able to relate to Laura S.'s experience with adding local foods to an already full schedule. "Probably the biggest challenge is that buying local tends to be less convenient and more work. Farmers' markets and the Fresh Stop are only open at very limited times of the week. Having an abundance of fresh food means it's necessary to commit to cooking and preparing it—lots of chopping, figuring out good recipes, and finding energy to cook consistently— before things spoil. Maintaining a garden, while rewarding, is also a lot of work, and there were many nights when I'd get home from work and wanted to let the weeds take over rather than go tend it. Also, local meats and dairy products tend to be significantly more expensive and our grocery budget isn't able to handle that now."

While we can't add extra hours to your week, there are many ways to economize on both time and finances to make local foods fit your family's needs.

STICKER SHOCK

Cost is commonly cited as an argument against buying local foods, and it is true that some local foods come with a higher price tag than their long-distance counterparts. Small local farms simply cannot always compete with highly efficient, highly subsidized agribusinesses. However, to put things in perspective, families in the United States spent just under 10% of their income for food in 2006, according to the USDA, the lowest percentage in the world. Other countries spend significantly more. Italians spend 18%, Filipinos 55%, and Tanzanians spend an astonishing 71% of their income on food.[34] Any premium that you pay for local food is still going to be a relatively small portion of your total food budget. It is also possible that in the not-so-distant future, as fuel costs continue to fluctuate, local foods will triumph in the price wars due to the mounting cost of transportation.

When making cost comparisons, it is important to compare apples to apples. Fresh, local foods can be more expensive at times, but if we compare them to high-priced health foods or convenience foods, local can still come out the winner. Rather than comparing high-quality local foods to the very cheapest big-box-store veggies or meat, try comparing them instead to foods of similar quality, such as those found at natural foods stores. Local will likely come out looking like a bargain.

Some people find that local foods are actually cheaper than comparable items at the grocery store. One young mother we surveyed wrote, "I can get local, free-range, and organic foods direct from the farmer cheaper than what I find at the grocery store. If the local foods are free-range and organic, my family benefits from foods that are highly nutritious, free of pesticide residue, and delicious." Sounds like a win-win situation!

HIDDEN COSTS

Cheap food isn't always cheap, in the end. Some foods carry a high cost to human health, farmers and communities, and the environment. As taxpayers, we all bear these costs when tax dollars

---

34   "The Influence of Income on Global Food Spending," USDA Agricultural Outlook/July 1997. www.ers.usda.gov/publications/agoutlook/jul1997/ao242e.pdf

clean up polluted rivers, subsidize unsustainable farming practices, and bail out bankrupt farmers.

Growing nutrient-rich food takes additional inputs, labor, and time, and often results in higher prices than the grocery store. Some of us are constitutionally frugal, though. We clip coupons, comparison shop, check unit pricing, and buy loss leaders. Fresh, local foods seem expensive and wasteful by comparison. But we need to take a longer view: while nutritionally dense foods may cost more pound for pound, what if we compare them vitamin for vitamin, or mineral for mineral? A customer who is a medical doctor's wife reminds me, "We either pay at one end of life or the other." We need to ask ourselves if we are willing to pay for our health up front or prefer to wait until disease sets in.

Ron and Mary M., who run an organic farm and CSA in Coshocton, OH, shared their perspective on the higher cost, in both time and money, of local and organic foods. "The cheapest food is corn-based, processed, and factory-made. We're conditioned to look for bargains, including food. But cheap food is expensive when you consider personal health and the health of farm and factory workers, environmental degradation, and subsidized fuel and transportation. Too-busy lifestyles encourage us to eat fast food and already prepared meals. It takes time to prepare local foods and it's easy to think we don't have that time. Advertisements lure us to processed non-local foods. We're used to getting almost any kind of produce at any time of year in the grocery store—that can discourage us from eating what's locally and seasonally available."

It is very difficult to estimate the environmental costs, in dollars, of industrial agriculture, but these costs must be borne by someone, and usually it is the taxpayer who ends up paying them. These costs are, in effect, a hidden subsidy paid out to agribusiness at our expense. They include the contamination of groundwater, rivers, and lakes by pesticides and fertilizers, damage to fisheries, drawdown of aquifers for irrigation water, health risks to workers and neighbors from toxic substances, noxious odors and flies, fuel usage contributing to air pollution, lack of species diversity, and so on.

Between $10 and $30 billion is paid out in direct cash subsidies to U.S. farmers and landowners each year. Over 90% of that money subsidizes just five crops—wheat, corn, soybeans, rice, and cotton. About a million people receive subsidies, but the largest producers receive by far the largest payments.[35] The $13.4 billion paid out in 2006 works out to roughly $44 for every person in the United States.

Most small farmers, on the other hand, and particularly those growing produce, do not receive subsidy payments. Since no one is helping subsidize their products, they may cost more up front. And as long as oil is relatively cheap, there are efficiencies of scale that large farms can take advantage of, which small farms do not benefit from. A small farm probably can't hire a crop duster to hit all of their fields, or buy the expensive, computerized equipment it takes to farm thousands of acres. But industrial agriculture is not healthy for the environment in many cases, as it encourages mono-cropping (which leads to a lack of species diversity and requires more chemicals), use of heavy equipment that compacts the soil, and shrinkage of rural communities as fewer and fewer farmers farm more and more land.

Sometimes you're just plain paying for higher quality. The grass-fed beef you purchase has as little as one-third as much fat as its feedlot counterpart, so when you cook up a pound of hamburger, you are left with more usable meat. Pastured eggs and meats have been shown to contain higher levels of omega-3s, vitamin E, CLAs, and other nutrients (see www.eatwild.com for a list of such studies). Food containing more nutrients lessens the need for vitamin supplements and should, over time, translate into healthier bodies requiring fewer doctor visits.

Along with higher quality often comes increased labor cost as more of the work is done by hand rather than by machines. The Amstutz family has been raising pastured turkeys on a small scale for the past few years. Several times a day, someone must take them food and water and move the pen to a fresh plot of grass. We purchase high-quality feed that is specially mixed for us at a local feed mill and do not get the volume discounts on feed or on the chicks themselves that a large operation would receive. But although our turkeys cost us more than the Thanksgiving specials at the supermarket, we feel that

35   Edwards, Chris. "Agricultural Subsidies," Cato Institute Website, June 13, 2007. www.cato.org/downsizing/agriculture/agriculture_subsidies.html

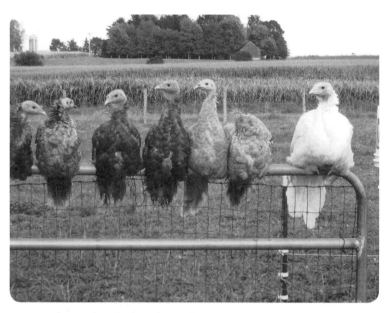

Bourbon Red and Blue Slate turkeys perch next to a Broad-Breasted White. Heritage turkey breeds, while slower-growing than commercial breeds, are known for their excellent flavor. A locally raised turkey makes the perfect centerpiece for a Thanksgiving meal that celebrates the bounty of the fall harvest.

the extra cost is worth it. Our birds taste wonderful, make a beautiful golden broth for gravy, and are not injected with water, fake butter, or any other additives.

Overall, we need to realize that when it comes to food, sticker price isn't everything. Finding out what is behind those costs may force us to take a long-term view of our choices and our world, to consider what it means to be a good global citizen. "We need to see purchasing locally made and grown products as an investment in our health, our community, and our country," says farmer James F. "Even if it costs us more initially, the long-term benefits need to be the focus. One person I know puts the food and medical columns together in her budget. Even though her food costs are higher, her medical costs are lower because of the quality food she is choosing. Educated consumers need to consciously choose purchases based on future implications, not just short-term frugality."

SAVINGS TIPS

Here are some money-saving tips from seasoned local foods shoppers to help you get started.

1. **Waste less.** Be intentional in using fresh foods in a timely manner. Dinner leftovers can be used as lunches or combined to make soups. Many cooks find they can get three meals from a whole chicken by eating it roasted one night, using leftover meat for casserole, curry, or stir-fry the next, and boiling the carcass to make a wonderful soup stock the third day. Leftover vegetables can be added to soup, stir-fry, or other combo dishes as well.

2. **Buy in bulk.** Many farmers offer attractive discounts on larger purchases. For instance, you can buy a quarter of beef, pork, or lamb for a fraction of the cost of individual cuts. You get all the good cuts too—you won't be limited to just ground meat. If your freezer isn't large enough to accommodate so much meat, consider splitting with friends or renting a freezer. You can also purchase large quantities of produce cheaply during peak season and preserve the excess by canning, freezing, or drying it (see chapter nine).

3. **Keep a pantry.** You can cut down on transportation costs by buying larger quantities of nonperishables when you find a good source, and again, you can preserve your own foods when they are plentiful. Don't have room? Perhaps you could store some things like grains and honey under your bed, desk, or stairs in plastic containers or convert part of another cupboard or closet to pantry space, even if it isn't in your kitchen.

4. **Eat more fresh, whole foods.** Learn how to roast a whole chicken, process fresh produce, and cook from scratch. Consider learning how to bake bread or make your own pasta. Your diet will be healthier without all the added salt and preservatives that are added to processed foods, and you get more bang for your buck when you buy whole potatoes rather than Tater Tots, or fresh green beans rather than canned. Even pizza, that perennial late night or family night favorite, can be both healthy and local when made with fresh ingredients like home-canned pizza sauce, local meats and cheeses, and a heap of seasonal vegetables. And splurging on a few high-quality ingredients like sea salt, freshly ground pepper, extra virgin olive oil, and fresh herbs can make ordinary meals taste gourmet.

5. **Combine errands or join a buying club.** Driving from farm to farm, or to distant farm markets, can pile on the miles. If you can find a nearby friend to carpool with or ask them to pick up items for you, you can cut down greatly on your transportation costs. In addition, some farmers offer buying club groups, where one person can pick up and distribute the goods and others will deliver weekly CSA boxes to a central location. If your farmer does not offer this option, perhaps you can offer to help organize it.

6. **Plant a garden.** We will cover this topic more thoroughly in chapter eight, but gardening can significantly reduce your food expenses. A two-dollar packet of seeds will yield more tomatoes or zucchini than you can possibly eat, and if you start with non-hybrid seed, you can save seeds for the following year and plant them for free. Yard and kitchen scraps make excellent compost and eliminate the need for expensive fertilizers.

7. **Eat less meat.** Consider using meat more as an accompaniment than a main dish, as many cultures do. Curries, stir-fry, jambalaya, soups, and casseroles all use relatively small amounts of meat in relation to the other ingredients. Using meat more sparingly will stretch your grocery dollars and is arguably a healthier way to eat. It is healthier for the planet as well—it takes 10-16 pounds of grain and a gallon of oil to produce a pound of meat by conventional methods, and even grass-fed meats require a lot of water, land, and other resources. Replacing some meats with grains, beans, and vegetables is a win-win situation.

8. **Look for seconds.** You can sometimes get fantastic deals on imperfect produce from farmers who can't otherwise market it at produce auctions, or even at the supermarket. The end of the season is another great time to find bargains—one local farmer sells his pick-your-own apples for just five dollars a bushel the last few days of the season.

Michelle Y., a research assistant, benefits from the imperfect produce grown at her place of employment. "I have access to 'unmarketable' produce from work that makes for great eating despite the imperfect appearance. I love golf-ball-sized potatoes for making stew, undersized butternut squash is perfect for a one-person serving, and tomatoes with minor blemishes are great for making spaghetti sauce," she writes.

9. **Consider it an investment** in your health, the health of your community, and the health of the planet. Perhaps you will sometimes end up spending more—but Americans are generally willing to spend more for quality (think $4 cappuccinos, $100 haircuts, leather-seated cars, and big-screen TVs). Why do we balk at buying quality food for our own bodies? We certainly spend lots of money on clothes, facial creams, and tanning to make our bodies look better superficially— why not invest in healthful foods that will make our bodies not only look better but feel better too?

Where did we get the idea that our food should be cheap? Sometimes in the supermarket, a young mother or father is in line in front of me. I stand there and watch them unloading a cart full of manufactured "food"—boxes of crackers and breakfast cereal, loaves of white bread, bags of snack foods, soft drinks and juice drinks, boxed dinners, and cans of Spaghetti-Os. The meat is hot dogs or bologna. When the cashier rings up their purchase the bill is substantial, but the actual nutrition in their cart, to my mind, is terribly inferior in quality. If that parent had spent the same money at a roadside stand and a bulk food store they would have plenty of fresh fruits and vegetables, some high-quality meat and cheese, and a grocery bag full of nuts, whole grains, and baking ingredients, and dried fruit to snack on.

We shouldn't expect to save money if we eat locally. Sometimes buying locally produced food costs substantially more per pound than if you'd bought it at Giant Eagle, but the environmental cost of that food is far more. For some reason we never count that! If you buy from local producers, you are also helping someone who is trying to be a good steward of the land. You might even be saving a small farm—which is important for the environment and for future generations.

One of the biggest challenges is the huge amount of time I spend with local, fresh food compared to when I just bought things at the supermarket. For instance, anything I harvest from the garden has to be washed and cleaned before use— everything needs to be taken from its original garden state to an edible table-ready product. This means you handle your food a lot more and spend time with it in a way you don't when you open boxes and bags from the supermarket. This also causes you to value your food and the work it takes to prepare it. Consider that dish of shelled peas you place on the table as a side dish with your meatloaf and mashed potatoes. The few small bags of frozen peas in my freezer represent an entire summer afternoon—and then some!

People who eat local foods have to learn to think of getting their food supply as family entertainment and an enjoyable adventure. Saturdays can be devoted to going to a farmers' market or traveling to a CSA or some local food vendor and then working together to plan meals. Ideally, the planning and preparation of food will be something the entire family shares in and not the sole responsibility of one person.

-Joanne L.

THE TIME CRUNCH

Buying local is certainly not always convenient; you generally can't make one stop at the supermarket to load up on local fruits, vegetables, grains, and meats. Additionally, when you begin cooking with more whole foods and give up the prepackaged meals, the reality is that food preparation is going to take a little longer. However, there are ways to make both the shopping and the cooking parts of eating local more efficient.

The hardest thing for me to adapt to in buying locally is the time it takes to travel to all the different stops. Vegetables from this stand, eggs and milk from this farm, fruit from another. Our world is just so fast-paced (not necessarily a good thing) that it makes it hard to find the time to skip the convenience of the supermarket.

When we lived overseas, everything we bought was local. There were no preservation techniques that could be used around the local open market that would allow food to be brought from too far. Just getting the food home before leaves wilted or meat spoiled was challenge enough by the time the haggling, boat transportation, and hauling up the hill had occurred. I miss it sometimes…

-Kelly S. and her husband are both nurses and realize the importance of eating well. Finding fresh local foods is one way they work at keeping their family healthy.

The other possible solution to the convenience conundrum is simply to reframe it. Look at the time spent shopping the countryside or cooking as entertainment, an investment in your health, or an education for your children. Visiting the farmers' market gets you out in the fresh air to stretch your legs, lets you develop relationships with farmers, and is a generally interesting way to spend a Saturday morning. By seeing your local food search as an adventure rather than an obstacle, your life will be richer. When you thoughtfully spend the time to purchase and prepare your food, you may learn to appreciate it more and to create new food-centered traditions in the process.

DEALING WITH SCHEDULES

Shopping for local foods is not generally one-stop shopping, unless you are blessed with a bountiful, year-round farmers' market. Even then, you may need to rearrange your schedule to arrive during peak hours. And sometimes it just won't work out. Lisa Z. found this out the hard way. "I've had the worst luck with getting eggs from my Amish neighbors," she says. "I've tried three times in the last couple weeks to get eggs; they weren't home, they were out of eggs even though the sign was up, and lastly, the drive was *way* too muddy! That's the frustration that comes with buying locally."

Both farmers and eaters need to make choices about keeping their lives and schedules balanced and those choices will directly affect the other group. Greater selection and longer hours make a farm store more appealing to the consumer but also mean extra commitment for the farm family. Sue S. is a former produce farmer who has learned to make trade-offs when necessary from both the perspective of a producer and a consumer. She wrote about some of the trade-offs she sees. "The less willing I am to accommodate the producer, the fewer sources I have to draw from. The producer who offers more products and longer shop hours is an easier draw for people, but that is not an easy thing to do as a producer without a lot of time, money, energy, and luck. If I have limited time and energy, where do I put my effort? I have to make decisions as to what is realistic for me and my situation and schedule. I may choose to be truly committed to local foods, but it will have to be with the knowledge that I will have to sacrifice some things (availability, convenience, time, expense) in order to gain the benefits (supporting local farmers, supporting local economy, freshness, nutrition)."

CONVENIENCE TIPS

1. **Combine errands** when possible, and see if you can find others to take a turn picking up items. By joining a **buying club**, you may only have to travel to the farm once in awhile, and someone else can pick up your order the other times. Or **join a CSA** and pick up a weekly basket of fresh foods either at the farm or at a pick-up point near your home.

2. **Stock up** on easily stored products when you make the trip for a special item. Lisa's family likes to buy cheese from a small local cheese factory, but it is too far away to justify a weekly trip. When we happen to be in the area, we buy about twenty pounds and freeze it for later use. Other items can be frozen as well—meats, butter, grains, etc. Fresh eggs will keep for weeks—much longer than supermarket eggs that may already be several days or weeks old when you buy them.

3. **Plan ahead.** Since you won't likely be able to just stop by the store every evening and purchase ingredients for dinner, planning menus in advance can help you to know what you will need for the week and you can arrange your shopping accordingly. *Saving Dinner*, by Leanne Ely, has seasonal weekly menus planned out with shopping lists included. I sometimes go through one of my seasonal cookbooks and make out a menu and grocery list for two weeks, then shop accordingly. We save these menus and reuse them the following year.

Learning a few basics and planning ahead can make fresh food into convenience food. Cook a cut of meat one night and use the scraps for soup the following night, chop all your onions or carrots for the week at one time, etc. Jennifer B., a mother of two young children, was initially unsure about the idea of cooking a whole chicken, but was very pleased with the results. "The idea of cooking a whole chicken was intimidating. With two small children, how could I possibly make something taste good without tons of preparation time? We ordered some pastured chickens from a local farm and they came with helpful recipes. I must say I did a pretty good job—prep work only took a few minutes and after a few hours, the chicken roasted to a nice golden brown and smelled wonderful. The meat was very tender, plus the leftovers made great enchiladas, soups, stir-fries, etc. We have been spoiled by good chicken!"

Another mother of young children said, "Local food tastes good. And I think we waste less because we've been really deliberate about obtaining it. While getting local food sometimes costs a bit more, I think it just as often costs less. Especially meat. And it keeps the money in the locale, which is really important in a struggling economy like northeast Ohio's."

4. **Fresh produce** can create gourmet meals but can also stand alone in simple dishes because the flavor doesn't have to be enhanced by fancy sauces, sugar, or salt. Many foods taste great raw and require minimal preparation—salads, a bowl of sugar snap peas, whole strawberries, etc.

5. The **slow cooker** is a great time-saver for the busy cook. By taking a few moments in the morning or the evening before to mix up a soup, casserole, chicken, or roast with vegetables, you can come home to a delicious, hot meal. Unfortunately, many of the slow cooker recipe books on the market rely heavily on processed foods, but they can still provide inspiration, and with some substitution of fresh ingredients, they can be a useful resource. For instance, rather than overly processed mushroom soup—the all-American food glue— use a homemade cream soup mix or white sauce. Canned vegetables can be replaced with fresh or frozen versions, and processed "cheese food" replaced with real, local cheese. See Appendix A for a delicious potato meal created with the help of the slow cooker.

"Convenience is the biggest barrier in my opinion; you don't have to plan ahead if you just eat at McDonald's all the time. Eating locally requires thought, which is just too much work for some people!" -Adam H., Amish farmer

Cooking with fresh, healthy ingredients definitely takes time and planning ahead. I'm learning to use my slow cooker more often on those days we know life will be hectic at suppertime. I've invested in a couple of slow cooker cookbooks and found recipes online. Roasts, stews, sloppy joes, pasta dishes, and soups are some of our favorites and

I'm always adding new things.

Unfortunately, during the summer when fresh produce is most abundant at roadside stands and local orchards, our time for cooking is slim. Children's sporting events, outdoor activities, and the fact that it doesn't get dark until late make it tempting to just grab convenience foods at mealtime. So I've worked at washing and cutting up veggies ahead of time to have a supply on hand for several days.

Since it's hard to find good, nutritious bread that isn't super expensive, I've learned to bake my own simple whole grain bread. I mix extra dough to freeze so it is ready to be baked whenever I need it. Plus baking bread always smells so good and warms up the house in winter. It takes time to do this extra cooking from scratch, but we are making a healthy diet and fitness a part of our lifestyle because I'm seeing how important it is to our family's health.

-Bonnie W. and her family have a full schedule that includes an intensive home remodeling project. They are thankful for abundant farm stands near their home. They have witnessed the positive effects on their family's health when they make wise food choices.

6. **Learn the art of food preservation.** While the actual process is time-consuming, a well-stocked pantry will provide you with your own local "convenience" foods later on. For example, one big batch of pasta sauce canned during peak tomato season makes for lots of quick pasta meals throughout the year. Canned vegetable soup or apple pie filling yield quick and easy meals, and dehydrated fruit makes for handy and healthy snacks. Frozen chopped green peppers or onions are great time-savers as well.

7. **Make a double batch** to use later in the week or for lunches, etc. If you're making homemade pizza, bake an extra one and put it in the freezer for a quick meal on a busy night. Soups, sauces, meats, and some kinds of casseroles freeze well and it's usually not any harder to make a double batch than a single one. Entire books have been written on the topic of making dinners for the freezer, most notably *Once a Month Cooking*.

8. **Find some like-minded friends** and start a supper club where each member cooks for the whole group one night per week and has meals delivered on the remaining nights. Trish Berg, who lives on a

family beef cattle farm and understands the juggling necessary with children's schedules, work, and family needs, has written a helpful guide entitled *The Great American Supper Swap.*

CONCLUSION

Cost and convenience can seem like steep hurdles to overcome when you begin buying local foods, but they are not insurmountable. By learning some simple money and time-saving tricks, you can turn your local food purchases into true bargains for your family's budget and health. Like most things, it all starts with a few small steps and tiny, manageable changes. As you add new skills and routines to your repertoire, you will find yourself conquering those hurdles.

THREE MEALS FROM ONE CHICKEN!

A pastured chicken may seem like a hefty investment at $2.50 per pound or more, but the frugal cook can easily stretch it into three satisfying meals. Not only does this make wise use of every part of the meat, it offers natural menu planning for the week.

Day 1: Sprinkle a 5-6 lb. whole, thawed bird with 2-3 T. chopped rosemary, 3 cloves of garlic, and salt to taste. Roast for 2½-3 hours at 325°.

Day 2: After the first meal of roasted chicken pieces, debone the remainder of the meat and use in a chicken and rice dish, chicken burritos, or a casserole.

Day 3: Cover the carcass and bones with water and simmer several hours with onions, celery, garlic, and herbs. Cracking the bones to expose the marrow and adding a splash of vinegar will help extract even more nutrition from the bones. The strained broth and remaining meat bits can then be used for a final meal of chicken soup.

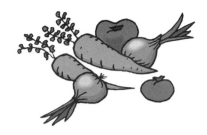

CHAPTER 8

In Your Own Backyard

Good gardening is very simple, really. You just have to learn to think like a plant.
-Barbara Damrosch

Local foods can be as close as your own patio. A simple container planted with parsley or basil, a few tomatoes in a flowerbed, or some productive raised beds can bring your food supply closer to home. Measuring the distance from field to table in footsteps rather than miles brings a new meaning to freshness and enriches your life with benefits beyond good food.

LESSONS FROM THE PAST

The local foods movement is actually a return to the way the world was before the advent of cheap oil and industrial-strength agriculture. In years gone by, local foods were the only option, with many families growing a sizable portion of their own food. The pioneers were dependent on their gardens to sustain them through the entire year. During the Depression, a garden was necessary to keep food on the table for many families. Victory gardens during World War II helped people survive the wartime shortages. "Recession gardens" are a growing trend in recent years as many families have planted gardens in order to lower their food bills.

Perhaps a nationwide return to backyard gardening will become a lifesaver for our environment and health today. Next time you drive by a subdivision, imagine what it would be like if all those acres of lawn were converted to gardens, and how many mouths they could feed. Consider how much oil we might save with less grass to mow and fewer food miles.

WHY GROW A GARDEN?

Fresh-cut herbs and just-picked tomatoes are only the tip of the iceberg. Agriculturalist and philosopher Wendell Berry shares this wisdom on the virtues of gardening: "I can think of no better form of personal involvement in the cure of the environment than that of gardening. A person who is growing a garden, if he is growing it organically, is improving a piece of the world. He is producing something to eat, which makes him somewhat independent of the grocery business, but he is also enlarging, for himself, the meaning of food and the pleasure of eating."[36]

For those who view local foods as cost-prohibitive, gardening can be an economical way to put fresh vegetables on the table. Many people feeling the pinch of high grocery bills are choosing to start a garden as one strategy to stretch their food budget. Morgan Taggart, an Ohio State University Extension agent in Cuyahoga County, estimates that gardeners can save their families $500-$1000 on their grocery bill in a backyard plot of only 20' by 20'.[37]

Wisely purchased seeds are a great investment; a $2 packet of lettuce seed can provide a season's worth of salad. Free amendments like shredded leaves, kitchen scraps, and leaf compost will improve even the worst soil on your lot. Additional savings are realized when you consider the time you spend in the garden as part of your recreation and exercise, reducing the dollars needed for entertainment and the gym.

Heirloom seeds are old-fashioned, non-hybrid varieties that have been grown and passed on for generations.

Others opt for gardening because the variety of vegetables available in the supermarket or even as seedlings at local greenhouses

---

36   Berry, Wendell. *A Continuous Harmony* (Harcourt Brace Jovanovich: 1972).

37   Kick, Chris, "Relieve Some Food-Dollar Stress by Planting a Garden," *The Daily Record*, 4/28/2008.

is limited. The lure of a pile of seed catalogs with their delectable descriptions is a powerful antidote to winter. Some gardeners may choose a certain tomato for its low acidity or high vitamin content. Others make choices based on taste and painstakingly locate seeds for delicate greens, specialty beets, or gourmet carrots that are not grown commercially because they cannot be mechanically harvested or have a limited shelf life.

In addition to our weekly CSA basket, we keep a small garden in our backyard. Being vegetarians, we like to have a variety of vegetables, which we have had a hard time locating at the regular grocery store. Some of our favorite vegetables to grow are leeks, beans for drying, and heirloom tomatoes. The dried beans are mostly for fun—the beans themselves are just so beautiful when you shell them, but it's hard to grow enough for many pots of soup. The leeks are easy to grow and wonderful in all sorts of soups and lentil dishes. We also enjoy growing different varieties of eggplants like purple- and white-streaked, Asian purple long, and Thai green eggplants.

The other big benefit of having a garden is being able to just go out and pick a few herbs when you need them. We have tried many varieties of basil along with oregano, dill, and unusual herbs like sorrel. There's nothing like going out into the yard, picking a giant, ripe, yellow tomato and some fresh leaves of basil and just putting them together for dinner.

-Susan L. is a college professor and mother of a young son. She and her husband share their gourmet backyard produce with the resident groundhog.

ADDITIONAL BENEFITS

In addition to putting fresh green beans and corn on your table, a garden can be good medicine. Many see the act of gardening as a stress reliever. The physical act of hoeing helps to dissipate angry feelings, and nurturing plants provides a sense of value and self-worth. "Garden therapy" programs are even becoming popular at nursing homes, jails and mental health facilities.

Another beneficial side effect of growing some of your own food is the natural workout that tending peas or cultivating lettuce provides. Hoeing and shoveling build muscles, and all that bending, walking, and lifting burns calories. As a bonus, these calories used to produce

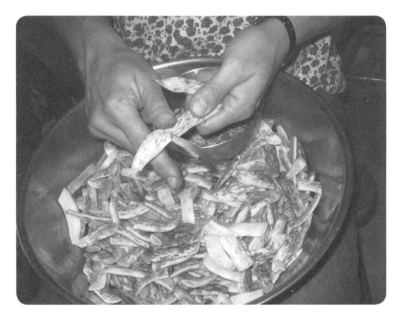

Fresh, healthful food is just a few steps away for the backyard gardener. Gardening is hard work, no question about it, but the rewards include free exercise, good food, a greener world, and often an abundance to share.

our food are not petroleum-based but from our own bodies. In the United States, most of us no longer need to expend any significant amount of physical energy to obtain our food. By coupling healthy food production with increased exercise, gardening offers significant benefits to our increasingly overweight society.

Ann H. finds working in the soil of her garden to be peaceful and tranquil especially after stressful days at work. She says, "Being in nature helps me stay focused on the important things of life. I also give up my gym pass during the summer since all the raking, pulling weeds, digging, pruning, etc. keeps my muscles toned and gives me a complete workout."

CREATIVE GARDENING METHODS

Gardening these days doesn't require an industrial-looking rectangular plot with plants arranged in rows like a marching band. Edible landscaping is an artful and creative way to incorporate vegetables into your flowerbed or yard. Raised beds neatly integrated into the landscape are increasingly popular and, when well managed, can be quite productive. Imagine lettuces of varying shades tucked into a flowerbed, herbs mingling with flowers, and climbing peas or beans crawling up a decorative trellis. Cheerful flowers like zinnias or sunflowers improve the appearance of the garden and, as a bonus, attract beneficial insects.

We live in town with a good-sized fenced yard. After starting with a small rectangular garden in the corner, we expanded the garden with an irregularly curved front, lined with rocks that blend in nicely with the flowerbeds. I am an informal landscape enthusiast, so most of our veggies are not in rows, but rather irregular little patches of lettuces, beans, onions, and tomatoes. Herbs are scattered throughout the flowerbeds and we included a few structures for vertical growth: stick teepees for sweet peas and runner beans and chicken wire frames for peas and cucumbers. We sprinkled grass clippings on the garden paths throughout the summer to add organic matter and to inhibit weed growth. We were pleased with the results—a more attractive garden, a better use of space, and less weeding. This year we plan to eliminate a bit more lawn as we add a curved bed along another portion of the fence.

-Corrie Y. is a reference librarian and mother of two preschool daughters. Her backyard is a work in progress as the garden expands and the lawn shrinks. They purchase meat, eggs, and crops that don't fit in their backyard from a local farm.

Innovative gardeners are full of tricks to reduce the labor required in their plots. Jim S., a veteran gardener in his upper seventies, still maintains raised beds that produce more vegetables than he and his wife can eat. His labor-reducing secret comes in the form of bags of leaves that the nearby village delivers to his home in the fall. His system is to put seeds on the ground, mulch with leaves, walk away, and return to harvest. This mulching method reduces the need for garden tools as well as the fuel to run those tools. The leaves also become the fertilizer for the next year's crop.

GROWING IN SMALL SPACES

Fortunately, owning a farm or even a substantial backyard is not a prerequisite for growing your own food. Many productive plots of food are appearing in tiny backyards and even on rooftops. By necessity, pocket gardens are common in many urban areas around the world and are now starting to catch on in the United States. Green Living reports that 15% of the world's food supply is grown in urban gardens, with some cities making impressive strides toward feeding themselves. Urban gardens in Hong Kong, the world's most densely populated city, provide about half of the city's vegetables and two-thirds of its poultry. In Moscow, around 65% of the population is involved in some form of urban gardening. In the United States, urban gardens are helping to rehabilitate low-income neighborhoods, providing jobs and fostering community relationships.[38]

Container gardening is becoming popular, especially for fresh herbs. You can grow tomatoes, peppers, and salad greens in containers on your patio for convenient, fresh harvesting. Try a large pot or trough, or even an old bathtub, for gardening on the back porch. Many gardening books list tips on watering, fertilizing, and cultivars that will stay well behaved in a small environment. Corrie Y. started her gardening career on the patio of the condominium where she and her husband lived as newlyweds. She found they had to water their potted tomatoes, peppers, and herbs heavily once a day and add fertilizer. Other than the year that the peppers kept disappearing because of the rabbits, they were quite pleased with the results of their patio jungle.

COMMUNITY GARDENS

You can still garden even if you lack acreage or if shade dominates your yard. Community gardens, where people divide a plot of land into sections so each one can have a small garden space, are

---

38   E Magazine. *Green Living: The E Magazine Handbook for Living Lightly on the Earth* (Plume: 2005) 17.

increasingly popular in urban areas. Laura, a social worker from a Cleveland suburb, told us about her first gardening adventure in a community garden a few blocks from their home:

> Originally started during World War II as a victory garden, the community garden has belonged to different groups and currently is reserved for seniors in our suburb of Cleveland. If there is extra space available, they allow younger folks like me to join in. There were 29 gardeners this year. My husband and I had a plot that was about 15' x 15' and grew green beans, radishes, lettuce, carrots, eggplant, broccoli, Hungarian wax peppers, green bell peppers, tomatoes, Swiss chard, and cilantro, and a few other things that didn't really produce. Our tomatoes were probably our most successful crop, and we were able to use them to make a great batch of salsa.
>
> The garden environment was a great place to learn, because you could stroll around and see the great variety of things people were growing and how they were growing them. In addition, there were a couple of very experienced gardeners who were more than willing to share their advice with me!
>
> *-Laura S.*

Community gardens are often located near apartment complexes, designated for seniors or other specific groups. To find a community garden in your area, check with the local extension office, town hall, or community center. If you are ambitious, locate a suitable vacant lot and approach city officials about transforming it into a community garden.

Another version of "community gardening" can happen when gardening neighbors band together to make their growing more efficient. Allyson L. and her husband used to be the only ones in their neighborhood to put out a garden. When the gardening bug bit several neighbors, they got together and decided to grow different crops and swap with each other. They also take some of the produce from their collective gardens to share with the less fortunate in their neighborhood.

GARDENING BASICS

To make your gardening efforts successful, some knowledge of gardening basics is essential. Excellent gardening books abound, local extension offices can provide resources, and older relatives or neighbors can be a valuable source of information and may be glad for your help as you gain hands-on experience. Keeping notes on planting dates, varieties, and harvest details will help you make adjustments in future years.

Site selection is a primary consideration and you will want to choose a level place that receives at least six hours of sunlight daily. Keep in mind that the closer you place your garden to your house, the more likely you will be to check it often, tend it easily, and be able to make quick harvests for cooking supper. It is essential to learn basic planting schedules and know which plants can survive frost and which will end up a pile of mush if the mercury dips below freezing. It is helpful to learn your region's planting zone (determined by frost date averages) to decipher planting dates listed in gardening books.

You may also want to research ideas for building up your soil since soil health is a key factor in producing healthy plants. Starting with a soil test (often free or low-cost through a county extension office) is a wise step so you know what amendments will be most beneficial. Double-digging and other deep cultivation methods can help to aerate a new plot of ground. If your soil is solid clay or otherwise beyond repair, there are also methods of creating new soil in a raised bed with a combination of peat moss, compost, vermiculite, and other amendments. (See the *Square Foot Gardening* book listed in the resource section at the end of this chapter.) For a small plot, some basic tools like a shovel, hoe, rake, and trowel are all that is needed to accomplish all of your earth-moving tasks. A watering can and hose, along with a source of unchlorinated water or rainwater, are helpful during dry spells.

Check out mulching options for retaining moisture and suppressing weeds. Consider fencing if rabbits, groundhogs, or neighborhood children threaten your tender seedlings. The wonders of compost, worms, companion plants, and beneficial insects are also worth investigating as you begin gardening. Learning the art of harvesting vegetables at optimum ripeness and various ways to cook and serve them will make your months of effort worthwhile.

Especially as you plant your first garden, it is important to remember that some crops will be a smashing success while others will seem a failure. However, no disappointment is a waste of time since you will learn valuable lessons along the way. A garden, like any worthwhile task, requires some discipline. Enthusiasm at planting time needs to continue through weeding, watering, pest control, and harvest. It does not need to consume hours each day, but frequent attention will keep weeds and problems to a minimum.

Kelly S. starts each gardening year with fresh energy and enthusiasm. She gets excited about new seeds sprouting and seeing the neat, weedless symmetry of the plot. Once the weeds come and keep coming, however, she confesses that she often wilts along with her unwatered plants. Then she is thankful for those who regularly raise fresh produce to sell.

If the weather is kind, the pests are minimal, and the weeds are under control, your garden may bless you with excess veggies. Abundances can be shared with neighbors (though be careful how much zucchini you leave on their doorstep!), families without time or space for a garden, or local food pantries. Stan K. finds great joy in sharing excess garden produce with neighbors and at church. Older folks appreciate being able to take home a single tomato, cucumber, or zucchini and Laotian friends are thankful for the green tomatoes Stan gathers for them at the end of the growing season to make special ethnic dishes. Extra tomatoes or beans can also be good incentives to learn food preservation techniques (see chapter nine) in order to extend the enjoyment of your hard work into the winter months.

BERRIES AND MORE

You may want to establish permanent plantings on your property to add variety to your garden. Perennials (plants that regrow each year without replanting) like rhubarb and asparagus are spring delicacies. Even small yards can house an assortment of berry plants that produce over a wide season; strawberries in late spring with blueberries and raspberries coming in summer through early fall. Grapevines and dwarf fruit trees also provide a good harvest from a small space. Be aware that some of these plantings take several years to mature and produce, so you need to consider how long you will live on your property, and whether you mind establishing plantings for future residents.

My love of growing trees comes from my father and grandfather. I started my organic mixed fruit orchard 14 years ago when we moved to a place where I knew we would be staying for a good long while. As finances allowed, I slowly added trees, mainly dwarf varieties. My orchard is tucked in by the side of my home and packed with apples, pears, peaches, native pawpaw, and cherry. With optimism and mixed success, I have also included Asian pear, persimmon, apricots, and plums. Our fruit does have some worms in it, especially some of the apple varieties, but we still have plenty for fresh eating, canning, and freezing.

Sometimes I get a bit frustrated when I see a squirrel dragging off one of my best pears or when the deer help themselves, but I remind myself that they were here first. Each tree has a beauty of its own and it is immensely satisfying for me to tend my orchard.

-Ann H. is the mother of three young adults and enjoys planting and harvesting on the rural property they share with her son's chicken flock and a pet pygmy goat.

BACKYARD LIVESTOCK

For the more adventuresome, backyard livestock can add enjoyment and additional fresh foods to your diet. Small chicken flocks, rabbits, or beehives can work even in town, and if you have a bit of acreage, you might consider some larger livestock like goats, sheep, or pigs. Raising animals requires commitment and a good knowledge of their food, water, shelter, and fencing needs, but it can be another great way to bring food production closer to home.

Learning about your town's local ordinances regarding livestock is an important first step. Appropriate housing and fencing is another prerequisite for a successful livestock project. Animals require daily care and depend on you for food and water, so consider who you can count on to do chores if you are out of town. If raising animals for meat, you also need to consider whether your family has the constitution to eat something they helped raise. 4-H programs offer good opportunities

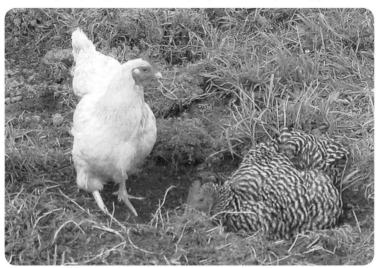

Free-range laying hens are free to express their "chicken-ish" nature by dust bathing and scratching for bugs. These hens lay eggs with deep yellow yolks that are high in CLA and omega-3s.

to introduce children to the art of animal husbandry. Even if you don't have the space for livestock, you could approach a neighbor with land and offer to help with chores in exchange for some eggs or meat.

One of the most rewarding experiences my family has had on our mini-farm was raising our first pigs. At first, we were a bit apprehensive about our decision. Would the pigs stink? Would we have enough food and space for them? Would we actually be able to eat them after raising them? Surprisingly, the pigs were a perfect fit. We gave them plenty of space so odor wasn't an issue and having enough to feed them was never a problem. Anything that didn't go to the compost pile went to the pigs: our old milk, whey, table scraps, and weeds—they really were like garbage disposals!

As for eating them...well, we haven't had a problem with that! The meat is the cleanest-tasting pork I have ever eaten, and we have a freezer full of it to last us through the winter. Not bad for a patch of land, organic pig feed, and some table scraps!

-Anna K., age 18, and her family maintain a very productive raised bed garden in addition to a menagerie of small livestock on their five-acre mini-farm.

A mini-farm isn't a requirement for raising livestock or making a significant contribution to the family pantry. Del M.'s family recently moved to a home on a one-acre lot and sought advice on how to use it to the fullest for food production. They added a fenced-in area for a few sheep and a run for laying hens plus space for a grape arbor, strawberry patch, and large garden. Amidst all this, there is still plenty of space for their children to play. Creative and efficient planning can turn even small lots into attractive and productive micro-farms.

CONCLUSION

Will flowerbed lettuce and tomatoes in patio containers be the victory gardens of our day? Could backyard chicken flocks once again supply families with eggs? At the least, these actions are steps toward making food more personal and appreciating the work that goes into producing a truly delicious meal. Backyard food production has the potential to keep families well fed and healthy in spite of rising fuel and food costs.

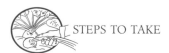 STEPS TO TAKE

1. Try growing herbs or salad greens in containers on your doorstep or windowsill.

2. Replace part of your lawn with a garden.

3. Offer to help a neighbor or friend in their garden or with their livestock and learn from them.

4. Investigate community gardening efforts in your area.

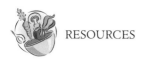

RESOURCES

1. Your local extension agent or 4-H club

2. *The New Square Foot Gardening* by Mel Bartholomew (www.squarefootgardening.com)

3. *The Vegetable Gardener's Bible* by Edward C. Smith

4. *The Edible Salad Garden* and others by Rosalind Creasy

5. *Barnyard in Your Backyard: A Beginner's Guide to Raising Chickens, Ducks, Geese, Rabbits, Goats, Sheep, and Cows* by Gail Damerow

6. *Food from Small Spaces: The Square-Inch Gardener's Guide to Year-Round Growing, Fermenting, and Sprouting* by R.J. Ruppenthal

7. Baker Creek Heirloom Seeds, http://rareseeds.com, (417) 924-8917

8. Johnny's Selected Seeds, www.johnnyseeds.com, (877) 564-6697

RECIPE FOR A BASIC KITCHEN GARDEN

A kitchen garden is designed for eating fresh and is ideally located near a kitchen door for quick harvesting. Here is a starter plan to make good use of a 4' x 8' space with planting dates geared for zone 6.

In early April or 5-6 weeks before last frost date:

Choose a day when ground is dry enough to be worked, because digging in wet spring soil will lead to hard, clumpy ground.

Make soil amendments, such as working in a 2" layer of compost.

Plant a 4' row of lettuce seed, a 4' row of mesclun mix or spinach seed, and a 4' row of radish seed with rows 6" apart.

You can begin harvesting fresh leaves for salad as soon as they reach 3-4". Radishes may be pulled as they reach eating size.

In mid-May, after danger of frost has passed:

Add three herb plants (parsley, basil, and rosemary or other favorites), a tomato, and a pepper plant. These can be purchased at a greenhouse or started indoors 4-6 weeks before planting out.

Tomatoes benefit from staking to keep fruit off the ground. Pick peppers green or after they change color a few weeks later. Pluck herb stems as needed once the plant is established.

Plant one hill of zucchini seeds and a 4' row of green beans (bush type or a pole variety if you have a trellis handy).

Once ripe, keep beans and zucchini picked so they will continue bearing. Small zucchini are great for stir-fries and larger ones shred easily for breads and other baked goods.

In late June, or when salad production is waning:

Plant four broccoli or cabbage plants where the salad was. These will be ready for fall harvest.

In many broccoli varieties, once the main head is harvested the plant will send out smaller side shoots that are also edible. So don't tear the plants out too quickly after harvesting! Cabbage heads can be harvested as needed and will tolerate frosty nights until the temperatures dip to the low 20s.

In August, when beans are done producing:

Plant more lettuce, spinach, and radishes, as space allows, for fall salads.

Mix up a quick salad dressing by shaking together 1/3 C. olive oil, 1/3 C. lemon juice, and 2 T. honey. Another version uses 1/3 C. olive oil, 1/3 C. balsamic vinegar, and 1 T. Dijon mustard.

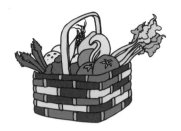

CHAPTER 9

Surviving the Off-Season

If we had no winter, the spring would not be so pleasant; if we did not sometimes taste of adversity, prosperity would not be so welcome.
-Anne Bradstreet

Just when we're getting spoiled by summer's abundance of fresh produce, those of us in northern climates are faced with months of snow and ice. Suddenly the only fresh things available in the supermarket have made the long trek from the tropics, and eating locally sounds impossible. The good news is, eating locally in winter is possible—but it does take some planning and foresight.

SEASON'S END

In our region, the roadside stands and many farmers' markets close their doors at the end of October, giving farmers a much-needed break to rest, plan, and dream about the next growing season. Thanksgiving offers a brief revival of local food offerings for the holiday table with some farms offering free-range turkeys, winter squash, sweet potatoes, and salad greens for one last feast before winter sets in. But what is available for those brave souls who decide to continue their local foods quest "beyond the turkey?" Large urban areas sometimes have indoor markets offering year-round winter produce, eggs, meats, baked goods, etc. Many winter cooks, however, will need to rely on either the supermarket or their own well-stocked pantries.

PUTTING FOOD BY

In years gone by, the main function of gardens was "putting up" food for the winter ahead. Shelves in pioneer homes groaned under the weight of rows and rows of canning jars. Strings of dried foods adorned the attic ceiling while crocks of sauerkraut and other ferments lined the basement along with crates of root crops. The family needed ample stores to make it through the lean months. Fortunately, most

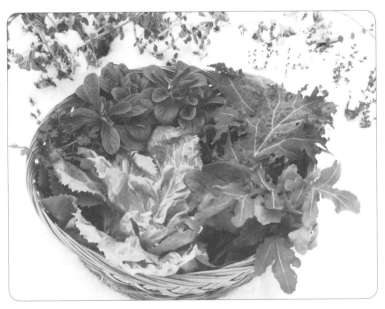

This salad was picked from an unheated greenhouse during an Ohio winter. Season-extending techniques make it possible for farmers and home gardeners in almost any climate to produce fresh greens year-round.

of us do not need to worry about going hungry if we haven't gone to all that work. However, those who want to continue eating local foods throughout the year can find helpful knowledge by looking to the methods of the past.

Although the art of food preservation seemingly went out of style when our grandmothers sold their canning jars at estate auctions, there has been a resurgence of interest by a younger generation wanting to preserve their own food and know its source. Many folks are relearning the secrets of canning, freezing, dehydrating, lacto-fermentation, and root cellaring.

Glenda Lehman Ervin of Lehman's in Kidron, Ohio reports, "We are seeing a trend in our store where the more high-tech people become, the more interested they are in low-tech items, which are the genre of the merchandise we sell. People want to get closer to their food source again. Eating lettuce and tomatoes from your own garden gives you more of a connection to your food source than a microwaved quick-pocket meal. Canning is the topic with the most hits on our website. Reducing your environmental footprint, nostalgia, and staying healthy are some reasons we think food preservation is again on the rise. Folks seem to be looking for simplicity in their fast-paced lives, and canning peaches, grinding grain, and making yogurt are ways they are finding that." The ever-increasing traffic at their "old-fashioned" store bears witness to this trend.

STOCK UP IN SEASON

Unless you grow your own, timing your shopping for quantities of produce to preserve is critical to making it affordable. Using the first-of-the-season tomatoes for canning, for instance, makes for pricey pizza sauce, while waiting until the peak of the season allows you to purchase large quantities at reasonable prices.

My current favorite resource is a farmers' produce auction about 20 minutes from me. It is largely stocked by Amish families who are raising produce for a living and bring it in their horse-drawn carts. The quantities are naturally larger and we do a lot of "putting away" of the items we get there. The prices can be very good and the quality is excellent. For a large family like ours, this can be a very good deal. Also, we notice that there are things available there that we do not see in other places, like strange, surreal squashes, unusual grape varieties, flowers, nursery plants; this makes it fun to go. Sometimes this means some "hanging around" while waiting for the lot we want, or it might mean going home empty-handed if the things we wanted went higher than we could pay...but it is always a fun trip.

-Andrea G. is a mother of five who is both a dedicated frugal shopper and healthy cook. Her children frequently join her in the kitchen to create nutritious meals.

Watching for peak season at the farmers' market or a produce auction is one of many ways to stock up. You might also plan a family outing to a pick-your-own berry or fruit farm, then go home to work together at canning applesauce or putting strawberries or blueberries in the freezer for winter treats. An ample freezer is helpful when purchasing meat in quantity such as beef by the quarter, a side of pork, or pastured chickens direct from the farm.

CANNING AND FREEZING

The most popular methods of preserving foods are canning and freezing. For good success, both require a careful knowledge of processes, times, and temperatures. You will also need to purchase some basic equipment to get set up. Many helpful books can get you started (see resource list) and an experienced friend or relative is a valuable resource if you are starting from scratch. Some produce, like chopped peppers or berries, may be put directly into containers and frozen. Others, like beans and corn, require a short blanching time

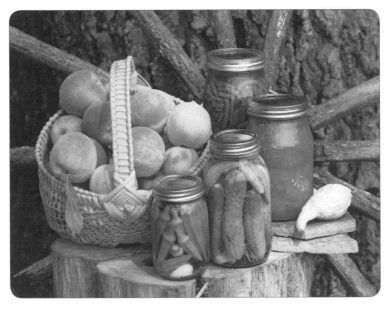

When produce is abundant, food preservation are an economical way to use up the bounty. Canning, freezing, dehydrating, and root cellaring are all ways your family can eat local around the calendar.

in boiling water or steam to retain quality in the freezer. Most frozen items are best used within a year.

Correct times and temperatures are vital to the quality and safety of your canned products. A pressure canner is a must for safely preserving low-acid items such as beans and meats while the water bath method is fine for most tomato products and fruits. Information from your local extension agent or a USDA website will inform you of current safety data. Once you learn the basics, there are many options to give you variety in winter meals—spaghetti sauces using a family recipe, salsas, pickles, even vegetable soup in a jar. Fruits canned as juice or jam make extra-special treats in the off-season.

Food preservation often requires large chunks of time, can be messy, and feels like a monumental task. Good planning and plenty of help will help you accomplish it smoothly. Canning and freezing may even become a summer tradition that creates new family memories.

My pantry shelves are not as full as my grandmother's probably were, but I do try to put away some key staples for my family to enjoy in the winter months, like green beans, tomato sauce, and sometimes applesauce. We have several different varieties of berries in our yard that we freeze in small amounts. Grass-fed meat purchased in quantity from a local farm also fills the freezer.

In our family, my husband really enjoys gardening in our small backyard, and I take responsibility for harvesting and preparing/storing food. Since my husband works a 9-5 job and I freelance as a violinist and mother four young children, I don't have time or energy to "put up" massive amounts of food, but we enjoy the feeling of accomplishing some of the food-raising ourselves. Plus it tastes good and puts me in touch with the lifestyle of previous generations in a way I would otherwise not appreciate.

When I have batches to process, I get help from family members and my husband, and try to do it in manageable chunks. I am not one of those people who stay up all night doing massive amounts of green beans all at once. Actually, my children enjoy helping me wash and pack green beans (I'll let them snap the ends, too). Then when my husband gets home from work, we put the canner on the stove while one of us is available to keep an eye on it.

A freezer is essential for us to eat well throughout the year, and ours is full of locally raised beef, chicken, and some frozen vegetables and fruits. It is enormously convenient for me not to ever have to buy meat at the grocery store; it's all just a staircase away in my home. And I know it is healthy and tasty, too! I've gotten really good at getting at least three meals out of one chicken (roasted first, then casserole, then soup with broth made from the bones and whatever meat is left) or one pot roast (slow cooker first, then vegetable-beef soup). This makes meal planning straightforward and the cooking simpler.

-*Amy G.*

DEHYDRATING AND LACTO-FERMENTATION

Dehydration is another method of preserving seasonal foods. Commercial food dehydrators are handy, but you can also dry food in your oven or use solar energy in dry climates. Foods dehydrated at low temperatures retain nutrients well. Apples and pears both dry nicely and make delicious winter snacks. Fruit leathers are extremely popular with children and healthier than the neon-colored, artificially flavored supermarket versions. Dried tomato slices retain excellent flavor and many other vegetables like celery and leeks also dehydrate well and taste good in winter soups. Dried foods can be stored in airtight jars or containers in a cool, dark place for several years. For more inspiration, we recommend *Food Drying with an Attitude* by Mary Bell.

Lacto-fermentation is another ancient food preservation technique. This original method for sauerkraut and other ferments uses Lactobacillus bacteria to create a high acid environment that preserves the food. Since no cooking is involved, the food retains enzymes that are lost during canning and other high-temperature methods. Most recipes call for a brine of salt, water and whey to start the anaerobic process.

Once finished, the jars or crocks of vegetables may be stored in the refrigerator or a root cellar. Though not complicated, lacto-fermentation takes some practice to perfect. A helpful tool for lacto-fermentation is a "Pickl-It" jar (available at www.pickl-it.com), a glass jar topped with an airlock system to eliminate the oxygen. Check out *Nourishing Traditions* by Sally Fallon to learn how to make your own artisan ferments.

ROOT CELLARING

Not all foods need to undergo involved processes like canning or blanching for freezing. Some crops can be simply stored in a place with proper temperature and humidity levels. Butternut squash can be stored in a cool (50-60°F) room and should keep until early spring. In the same climate, sweet potatoes individually wrapped in newspaper will last several months as well. Place onions and garlic in a mesh bag and hang in a dark place at room temperature. If you are fortunate enough to have a cool, damp basement room, you can easily store crates of potatoes and cabbages. Turnips, beets, carrots, and even leeks will keep well in this root cellar environment if stored in buckets of sand or sawdust to prevent dehydration.

Mary G., a business analyst, finds this quite doable, even with limited space. "I live alone, but grow and can and freeze as much as I am able," says Mary. "Last summer I borrowed a 200' row from a friend and was able to produce quite a few green beans, edamames, and beets. I don't have a basement or root cellar, but save onions, garlic, apples, and winter squash in my attached garage."

IN THE GARDEN

If you are a gardener, season-extending tricks can stretch your harvest into the winter. By simply staggering plantings of lettuce, green beans, and other crops, you will be able to eat fresh produce over a longer time than a single planting allows. Cold frames are a common sight in many European countries and are gaining popularity with U.S. gardeners. These structures can be as simple as plastic barrel halves or an old window set on cement blocks to protect spinach, lettuce, and other cold-hardy greens. Another way to continue eating from the garden during the cold months is to cover root crops like carrots, beets, and turnips with a thick layer of leaves or straw and dig as needed.

I (Karen) would much rather spend my summer days outdoors in my garden than in a hot kitchen, working over a canner to preserve food for winter. So I first looked at how I could extend my garden seasons and started doing more succession plantings (beans, corn, lettuce) so we could eat fresh longer. After reading books by Eliot Coleman, an innovative organic gardener from Maine, I was inspired to try a cold frame for salad greens. I figured if he could do it in Maine, then surely it was possible in Ohio. That experimentation has resulted in our family having access to fresh salad greens all winter long the past eight years. Stretching our growing season has reduced the need to have the pantry filled to the brim by the end of summer and I get to do what I really enjoy—dig in the garden.

There are other innovative ways to garden indoors through the winter. Herbs such as parsley and rosemary grow nicely by a window and some people grow salad and more under fluorescent lights. Sprouts are another popular health food that you can grow right in your kitchen to supplement your winter produce needs. Radish, alfalfa, mung bean, and broccoli seeds are packed with nutrition and will sprout in less than a week in a simple glass jar with regular rinsing.

OTHER LOCAL OPTIONS

As we learned to eat seasonally, we began to notice options in the winter that we never paid attention to before—parsnips, leeks, strange squash, endive, and more. Meanwhile, as demand increases, we are seeing more options for purchasing fresh foods close to home in the colder seasons. Some CSAs now offer winter shares that include fresh greens and root crops kept in storage. Hothouses and high tunnels present new options for local year-round food production. High tunnels are basically giant unheated cold frames (usually constructed of hoops and plastic), which can be used to grow winter greens such as spinach, lettuce, and Swiss chard and get a head start on summer crops. Several state universities, including the Ohio State University research facility in Wooster, Ohio, are involved in research and training for commercial high tunnel production to develop year-round food production techniques. Other items like dairy, meats, and eggs should be accessible in the winter months as well.

Local Roots Market and Café in downtown Wooster, Ohio is

building on the success of the city's outdoor farmers' market to offer a year-round source of local foods. Farmers either add their products to the store's shelves or list them on the website. Shoppers can select from the array of local products at the retail store or create their own custom online orders. Future plans include a commercial kitchen where members can produce value-added foods such as salsa and jams, a butcher shop, educational seminars and more. Increased consumer demand may well encourage more area farms and markets to begin offering winter options.

Jessica Eikleberry started as a consumer members of the steering committee and later became the market manager. She writes, "My family got involved in local foods initially for personal health reasons but quickly saw it wasn't that easy to find the products we were looking for. You hear about food deserts in inner cities, but here we were, surrounded by cornfields and not able to find the fresh food we wanted. We knew there was demand for local foods from people like us—busy people with money to spend and the desire to eat local but no time to produce their own food. With Local Roots, I am excited to be a part of something that connects the many farmers in our area to consumers like me. I love how easy it now is to fill my shopping bag with local produce all year round!"

AT THE GROCERY STORE

Even if you haven't taken the time to preserve your own foods and there are no winter farmers' markets nearby, you can make choices at the grocery store to keep in step with the seasons. You can still look for locally produced meat and dairy products when your produce options are limited. Asking your grocer to stock local apples, root crops, and winter squashes through the winter months may help increase your choices. Lori S.J.'s family commitment to becoming more conscious about food choices led them to avoid buying tomatoes, peppers, and cucumbers in the grocery store during the winter months. They do buy carrots, squash, potatoes, and apples in the winter and find that limiting their fresh produce helps to focus on the seasonal nature of food items. Even if you can't find much local food in the winter, eating seasonal food is a good first step.

CONCLUSION

While eating locally in winter can be a challenge in northern climates, it is not impossible. With careful planning and preparation, winter meals can be as satisfying and nourishing as any other season's meals. Training yourself to eat seasonally and learning the skills of food preservation will ensure that you can eat locally and eat well— even in the dead of winter.

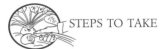

STEPS TO TAKE

1. Research and learn about food preservation methods. Ask an experienced person to let you help when they can or freeze produce.

2. When produce is abundant in your garden or at the farmers' market, buy extra to preserve for the winter—tomatoes, butternut squash, peppers, green beans, etc.

3. Try some season-extending tricks in your garden, like succession planting or cold framing.

4. Avoid buying clearly "out-of-season" items in the grocery store, such as tomatoes and cucumbers in January in northern climates.

RESOURCES

1. *Four Season Harvest* by Eliot Coleman

2. *Saving the Seasons* by Mary Clemens Meyer and Susanna Meyer

3. *Ball Blue Book,* www.freshpreserving.com

4. Your local extension agent (see www.csrees.usda.gov/extension or look in your local telephone book to locate an office)

5. Lehman's ww.lehman's.com. Helpful articles, a blog and product information. Call (888) 438-5346 for a catalog.

NO MORE ROTTEN TOMATOES

Home food preservation is an economical and healthful way to store a bountiful harvest of fruits and vegetables. It is a foolproof way to keep your table filled with local foods beyond your region's growing season.

Tomatoes are a popular and prolific item in many kitchen gardens; however, they are only available fresh picked a few months out of the year. We'll use tomatoes as an example and demonstrate three ways you can preserve them to enjoy in meals throughout the year.

1. FREEZE THEM.

Whole tomatoes can be washed, stemmed, and frozen whole in an airtight bag or container. Some people prefer to skin the tomatoes before freezing but they freeze equally well with the skins on. When you are ready to use them, simply pull out a few and thaw as needed to toss in a soup, sauce, or pasta.

Freezing is also a good way to preserve tomato sauce or paste, spaghetti and pizza sauces, tomato juice, etc. Simply cook according to recipe and freeze in plastic freezer boxes or other containers. Be sure to label your containers with the contents and the date—you likely won't remember what was in those containers come March. If you have the freezer space available, this method is considerably faster than canning.

2. CAN THEM.

There are a myriad of ways to can tomatoes and many families have signature recipes for things such as salsa, pizza or spaghetti sauce, tomato or vegetable soup, juice, sauce, paste, and whole or diced tomatoes. To get started you will need canning jars, lids, and rings, a water bath (a pot large enough to completely immerse the jars) or pressure canner, and a pair of tongs for lifting the jars out of the water. If you are juicing the tomatoes, you will additionally need some kind of a strainer (i.e. a food mill, Victorio strainer, or KitchenAid strainer attachment).

The basic steps to canning are sterilizing your jars and lids, preparing the fruit or vegetable, filling the jars, and processing them in the water bath or canner. Once the jars are removed all lids should "pop" and be sealed tight. Canned items are best stored in a cool, dark place like basement shelving.

There are some risks to home canned foods, which are easily avoided by using proper sterilization techniques and processing times. See the Ball Blue Book, USDA information, or your county extension office for safe and reliable canning information.

3. DEHYDRATE THEM.

Sun-dried tomatoes are an expensive gourmet item, but you can make your own easily and cheaply. Simply slice tomatoes in half lengthwise (small, meaty tomatoes like Romas work best, but any tomato can be dried) or in ¼" slices if larger, and lay on a tray. Sprinkle lightly with salt. Dry them in the sun, an oven, or a food dehydrator.

If you dry them outdoors, be sure to cover with clean cheesecloth or netting to keep the critters away—but don't let it touch the tomatoes. Bring them in at night so they don't absorb the dew. This method will take a number of days, depending on weather conditions.

The oven method is similar, except that it will only take a few hours rather than days. Set your oven to no higher than 140°, and prop the oven door open a few inches. Check frequently and remove when tomatoes are dry but still soft and pliable.

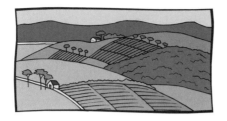

CHAPTER 10

Dining Out Closer to Home

We may live without friends; we may live without books,
But civilized men cannot live without cooks.
-Edward G. Bulwer-Lytton

Once you've gotten accustomed to the flavors of local foods at your kitchen table, you may want to look for ways to eat local away from home as well. In this chapter, we'll look at restaurants and caterers specializing in serving local, seasonal foods and explore ways to bring those foods to schools, institutions, and even fund-raising meals.

LOCAL FOODS IN RESTAURANTS

One early February day, the authors enjoyed creamy broccoli soup made with local dairy products, a mushroom tart prepared from mushrooms from a nearby mushroom farm, a corned beef and cabbage sandwich using local beef, gourmet salads with some greens from a hothouse in the next town, and other treats at the South Market Bistro. The Bistro is a local eatery under the direction of chef Mike Mariola and located in a renovated downtown building with Old World flair. The Bistro was established in 2002 with the goal of providing sustainable cuisine. According to their website, sustainable cuisine means preparing and consuming food with maximum respect for the environment and the health of our society as a whole. South Market Bistro uses the freshest local ingredients whenever available to support local farms, changes its menu with the seasons, and chooses organic ingredients whenever possible to support their concept of sustainable cuisine. During the peak summer months they are able to source 75-85% of their ingredients locally; during the winter those numbers scale back to half that amount. The other diners eating the day we visited were a diverse group—business executives, older women, a single man with a newspaper, and several couples along with casually dressed college students. Mike noted that his patrons are a loyal bunch, some returning because they appreciate good-tasting food, others because they like the idea of eating food grown locally.

More and more restaurants are featuring seasonal menus and sourcing foods locally rather than through giant food suppliers. The spectacle of a chef perusing the farmers' market with a wagonload of produce in tow is an encouraging sign that something good is cooking nearby. You can locate a local foods restaurant near you through Internet searches, word-of-mouth advertising, feature articles in cooking sections of your city newspaper, or even by asking vendors at a large farmers' market if they supply any nearby restaurants.

LOCAL FOODS RESTAURANTS FOR ALL BUDGETS

Some of the best seasonal restaurants are chef-owned and upscale, which can put them out of reach for the average budget. However, some moderately priced establishments and even some national chains are adding local options to their menus.

Ed and Denise Mack had a combination of experience in restaurant management and as farmers' market vendors. Prior to opening the Barn Stone Café, they owned a franchise restaurant and were involved in the local farmers' market. Selling their farm produce and baked goods at the market let them experience firsthand their customers' positive response to fresh, local foods. They felt that opening a restaurant offering locally produced items might be something area residents would appreciate but didn't think their community was ready for an upscale eatery. Their menu offers both a general section with soup and sandwich offerings and a section featuring local foods such as beef, chicken, salad greens, herbs, and produce in season. Denise notes that there has been extra driving time and cost involved in sourcing the local foods in addition to the challenge of getting patrons to try new dishes. However, the benefits of knowing that the ingredients are fresh, high quality, and beneficial to the local economy make their efforts worth it.

Alan K. is a market gardener who supplies gourmet salad mix to a small diner in his town. Alan shares, "One week our supply was short, so with permission I supplemented the order with head lettuce from another grower. I got a call from the owner saying that next week she wanted "our greens" because she noticed more uneaten salad coming back and less salad was being ordered. Through this experience we both learned the value that superior quality, gourmet produce can have for the restaurant business." Another food establishment promoting "local" is The Farmer's Diner in Quechee, Vermont. The restaurant's slogan is "Food from Here" and their goal is to spend 70¢ of every food dollar within 75 miles of the restaurant. Their focus is serving high quality but affordable food for working-class customers. Owner Tod Murphy has a vision of creating a chain of such restaurants with each region having a central butcher, dairy, and other processing facilities.

Other small, family-owned diners partner with small producers to the benefit of both and while some may only incorporate a few locally purchased ingredients, customers still notice. Cindy S.'s favorite pizza place in her hometown recently moved to a big, new restaurant. They had used sausage from a local butcher for years on their sausage pizza, her favorite. With the opening of the big restaurant, some large meat producers tried to get them to change to their brand of sausage. The owner said, "No thanks!"

Even some national chains are jumping on the local foods bandwagon, although the logistics get more complicated due to volume and sanitation standards. Chipotle Mexican Grill is leading the way in adding local foods such as lettuce, onions, and peppers to their menu. The chain has pledged to use a set amount of seasonal local produce at each of their more than 730 restaurants nationwide, sourcing it from small and mid-sized farms within a 200-mile radius.[40] Some question whether a corporate food chain fits in the local food economy, but these partnerships also open the door for local foods to go mainstream.

---

40 Tsai, Catherine. "Chipotle to Use More Local Ingredients," *New York Daily News*, June 18, 2008.

OTHER DINING OPPORTUNITIES

For several years Monique T. kept a busy catering schedule of cooking for upscale parties, weddings, and gatherings and delivering gourmet vegetarian meals two days a week to clients. Local foods were the backbone of Monique's meal preparations. She was both a regular vendor at the farmers' market with her gourmet granola and a frequent shopper, with her menus for the upcoming week in hand. She collaborated with a local farmer to provide some of the specialty greens and vegetables such as baby bok choy, mesclun mixes, and

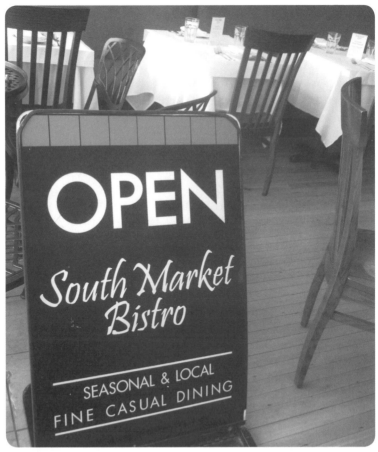

The South Market Bistro in Wooster, OH uses sustainably grown, local foods to create delicious gourmet meals. Local foods restaurants are increasingly popular, making it easier to eat local away from home.

herbs that she used to create dishes that sport fancy French names and highlight the season's best.

Another unique dining opportunity here in Amish country is the chance to eat in the home of an Amish family. The Weaver family hosts 25-30 tour groups each year for home-cooked meals in their Amish home. Several foods on the menu are raised right on the Weavers' farm: grass-fed beef from their Limousin cattle herd, abundant potatoes from their field, plus corn, tomatoes, peppers, beans, lettuce, and other seasonal vegetables from their garden. Older daughters decorate the tables with vases of flowers picked from the immaculate flowerbeds, and if asked, they will sing for the guests following the meal. Guests appreciate knowing they are eating a meal with ingredients grown right on the farm. One group of international students ate the bowl of homegrown creamed corn dry and commented on how good even the water tasted! Currently, each menu is still decided mainly by tour group guides, but the Weavers are exploring offering their own menu featuring all locally grown foods, many organic, to expand their business to other interested groups.

The Weavers' approach is a breath of fresh air compared to a statement we heard at a food and farming conference in our area several years back, when an Amish farmer commented how sad it is that there are so many "Amish" restaurants nearby and so little of the food served actually comes from Amish farms.

CREATIVE SOLUTIONS

Dining experiences that include local foods are wonderful, but they can be a strain on the pocketbook and may not be accessible to everyone. The Geiser family's taste buds have become spoiled with the good food we raise, and eating out has become more of an expensive disappointment than a pleasant night out. So we've come up with some creative solutions to satisfy both our palate and our budget. To celebrate our August anniversary, my husband and I started hiring friends to cook and serve us food from our farm in place of eating at a restaurant. One year we provided a sirloin steak and basket of garden vegetables and were served a scrumptious bulgogi in the dining room of one of our produce customers who enjoys cooking (see Appendix A for recipe). Another year, my Mexican aunt was visiting and gave us a list of the fresh ingredients (chicken, tomatoes, tomatillos, garlic, and other garden goodies) she needed to create a Mexican meal for our anniversary. Along with some foods local to her, like dried black peppers and tortilla corn, she created a feast to savor and remember.

Another thing we've done when we can't afford to eat out is to create "restaurant" meals at home. Most often, this is a Friday or Saturday supper that we spend extra time preparing and serve at a carefully set table. Sometimes we get our own grass-fed steaks out of the freezer or roast a pastured chicken, but it could mean splurging on another local ingredient. One night I came home with three live trout from a nearby fish farm. That made for a memorable meal preparation and a tasty meal.

EATING LOCALLY ON THE ROAD

Eating local while traveling can help you experience the flavor of a place more fully. Rather than refueling at a fast food joint, the

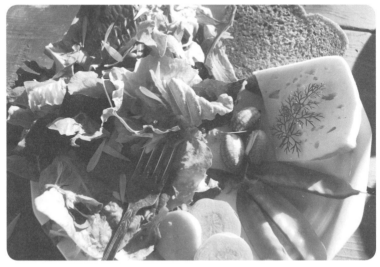

Simple, homegrown fare can be both beautiful and delicious when freshly picked and arranged with care. When eating out is not an option, high-quality ingredients and a little extra time can replicate a restaurant-style meal at home.

Amstutz family tries to find something unique to the area, even if it's just a family diner that serves local specialties. We've eaten conch fritters and key lime pie in Florida, grits in Georgia, waffles topped with fresh marionberries in Oregon, and pigeon peas and rice in the Bahamas, to name a few memorable meals. As we look back on those trips, we remember those meals as highlights.

Another thing we do, particularly for lunches, is to look for roadside stands or farmers' markets, buy some seasonal produce, a loaf of bread and some cheese, and make our own quick meals. On shorter trips, we generally just take along some local or homegrown lunch or snacks to munch along the way. This saves us the time and expense of eating out.

Most of our trips are to visit relatives or friends, so we typically stay in a home with meals prepared for us and with hosts who have those automatic connections with the local area. Sometimes I take along food from our home, like milk or yogurt, or produce from our garden or market. I enjoy visiting the local farmers' markets in the town where we stay and often buy food to make a meal for our hosts and sometimes more to take along home. Another resource we have used on trips is *Healthy Highways* by Nikki & David Goldbeck. This book gives state-by-state information on healthy restaurants and grocery stores, along with directions, hours, contact info, etc. Neither my husband nor I prefer fast food restaurants (though our girls do!) so we have explored several of these stores/restaurants on our travels, even though they are generally further off the highway.

-*Kris S.Z.*

LOCAL FOODS IN INSTITUTIONS

Most institutions that provide food service rely on weekly deliveries from national food suppliers. There are many obstacles to sourcing large quantities of local foods on a consistent basis, but some colleges are responding to student requests for a more sustainable diet.

Located in agriculturally rich Knox County, Ohio, Kenyon College is making intentional efforts to incorporate local foods into their dining services. Their "Food for Thought" program has brought awareness to food issues on campus throughout the disciplines for over a decade and was the impetus for bringing local foods to student tables during the school year.

The initiative began in 2004 with a couple of meals featuring local foods and has escalated to the point where over one-third of food purchases are now locally sourced. These include whole animal purchases (an average of 10 per week) procured from farms only 15 miles from campus, dairy products from family operations less than an hour away and grain products grown and milled in a neighboring county. Fresh produce comes from student-run gardens, over twenty local growers and the nearby Owl Creek Produce Auction. Apples, potatoes, jam and honey are sourced within a 20-mile radius.

Students gain greater connection to their food sources through on-farm internships and the sustainable agriculture curriculum. By virtue of increased sales, local farmers and food producers are better able to start, sustain and grow their livelihoods and businesses.

Intensive initiatives like this are certainly not without their struggles, as food procurer John Marsh can attest. He faces the challenges of dealing with the counter-cyclical nature of the academic year with the growing season and satisfying the cosmopolitan tastes of a couple thousand students transplanted to a rural village. When the Kenyon students got a taste of real broccoli, they doubled their broccoli consumption, but Marsh was unable to procure enough to keep up with the dining hall demand. "This is not uncommon," he says. "I am learning to better predict the consumption patterns of the students when we introduce fresh, locally grown and prepared food. Typically, what we see is a spike and then a tapering off at levels usually double or triple over the conventional equivalent for a particular item. I chase after demand every year. This is one of the most exciting and gratifying parts of my job and I love seeing students revel in the discovery and enjoyment of real food."

Institutions of higher education provide a natural seedbed for this type of program due to the activist nature of young adults, available funding and devoted staff. It can be a struggle, however, for cooks at the elementary and high school level to incorporate fresh, local foods into their menus. Even if they'd like to offer these kinds of foods, school cooks are often hamstrung by paperwork, government regulations, and extremely tight budgets. Some schools are responding by adding gardening to their curriculum and growing a portion of their own produce. Others have found creative ways—grants, budget tradeoffs, fundraisers, etc.—to raise the extra funds needed to provide students with more fresh, locally grown foods, and have found that kids respond positively, choosing to purchase lunch more often, wasting less food and even paying better attention in class.

Health care institutions are another natural place to initiate cafeteria changes to include healthful local foods. In 2009, the Wooster Community Hospital added a one-acre sustainable garden to its campus. Hospital patients and employees now enjoy the fruits of this garden in the hospital cafeteria. Stories like these are encouraging and perhaps they will inspire other institutions to take similar steps.

FUND-RAISING MEALS

Planners of fund-raising meals for churches or charities often rely on a shopping trip to a wholesale club, but could easily incorporate seasonal foods purchased locally into the menu. If transforming the entire menu feels overwhelming, start with just one dish created from local foods. By simply adding local hamburger to the spaghetti sauce or featuring a locally grown salad (and by making it known to your customers), you will make a statement that this meal is special. If there are any farmers in the group, they may be happy to contribute food as their donation to the event or in exchange for some advertising. Seasoned farmers' market patrons might be willing to help with menu planning around what is available and do the shopping. Even the decorations are something to consider sourcing locally, whether it be flowers from gardens of group members or fall pumpkins from a nearby farm. Guests are bound to notice the difference in the meal and that may prompt them to donate even more generously. By purchasing local ingredients, your benefit meal will not only benefit its intended recipients, but a local farmer or small business as well.

One church in our area hosts an annual Maple Syrup Festival to raise money for missions. Church members tap trees and boil down the sap to produce their own maple syrup. Others purchase a quantity of pork and spend an evening stuffing sausages. They then serve a breakfast of homemade pancakes (using local eggs), maple syrup, and sausage, and sell any leftover syrup. The meal is now an annual tradition that the community looks forward to, and is quite successful in generating contributions.

CONCLUSION

Dining out with local foods may take some detective work since many of these restaurants are small, grassroots operations. Some are a bit pricey, making them only special-occasion destinations for ordinary folks. However, as demand increases and more innovative chefs and restaurateurs hit the scene, restaurants offering local foods may become easier to find, with options to fit every budget. In institutions and fund-raising situations, your requests and offers to help can make more local fare a reality and can be an excellent opportunity to introduce others to the many benefits of eating closer to home.

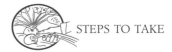 STEPS TO TAKE

1. Find out what restaurants in your area serve local foods and give them your business.

2. Talk with the food service providers at your school or place of work and request they try to obtain some of their menu items from local sources.

3. When in a "conventional" restaurant, choose foods that are in season.

4. Use your newfound local foods purchasing savvy to help make your next fund-raising meal extra special.

 RESOURCES

1. *Lunch Lessons: Changing the Way We Feed Our Children* by Ann Cooper and Lisa Holmes. www.lunchlessons.org/index.html

2. *Roadfood: The Coast-to-Coast Guide to 700 of the Best Barbecue Joints, Lobster Shacks, Ice Cream Parlors, Highway Diners, and Much, Much More* by Jane Stern and Michael Stern. www.roadfood.com (lists memorable local eateries along the back roads and highways of America)

ON THE ROAD AGAIN

Living as we do in the land of Swiss cheese and bologna, travel food for our family is often a hunk of locally made cheese, slices of cold meat, crackers, cut-up carrots or other fresh veggies, and seasonal fruit (apples, grapes, etc.). Other times it's homemade bread with peanut butter and homemade strawberry jam. Home-canned items pack well in the cooler; jars of peaches, pears, salsa, pickles, etc.

If we're eating in the car, I toss in cloth napkins and some smallish plastic containers for the children to hold their food in. Otherwise, we pack picnic items and eat at a rest area.

If we're staying overnight somewhere, we like to bring along a bottle of milk and a bag of granola, or yogurt and fruit, for a quick and easy breakfast. Most hotels have ice machines so it's not hard to keep food chilled in a cooler for a few days. With a large family, we've found it is often worth a few extra dollars to get a suite with a kitchenette—we easily make up the difference in cost by cooking our own food instead of eating out every meal.

For dinner, we like to eat out at a unique restaurant of some kind, featuring either local or ethnic cuisine. If that were not an option, however, it would not be difficult to pack a container of frozen soup or casserole to heat up.

Our family enjoys camping during the summer months, and we try to eat local when we camp as well. We bring along locally grown meats, potatoes, and veggies to make "hobo dinners" and grill some of our own chicken, bratwurst, and even sweet corn when it is in season. The ears are delicious soaked in salt water and then roasted in their husks. Fresh fruits and veggies such as green beans, sugar snap peas, carrots, and green onions are nice to have along. If we camp somewhere coastal, we usually buy some fresh-caught fish (or catch some ourselves!) to fry up for a meal as well.

Often we are able to find a little produce stand near the campground and pick up a watermelon, strawberries, or whatever other fruit is in season. One year we were lucky enough to be in Michigan at the peak of cherry season, so we ate fresh cherries until our faces were sticky and our bellies full.

Eating local on the road takes some extra planning, but the results are not only healthier than fast food options but cheaper and tastier as well. We'll take Old McDonald's Farm over yet another stop at McDonald's any day.

-L.A.

CHAPTER 11

Flowers: Going Beyond Food

If you have but two pennies in the world, spend one on a loaf of bread and the other on a lily.
-Chinese Proverb

W hat better way to take pleasure in a meal of fresh, local foods than with a centerpiece of colorful flowers? Their beauty provides a feast for the soul as we nourish our bodies with good food. Yet flowers, like our food, are a global commodity. It is worth investigating their origins and seeking out local sources for the blooms that adorn our tables, lapels, and celebrations.

THE MODERN FLOWER INDUSTRY

The language of flowers can express joy, sympathy, love, apology, and so much more. It is big business - U.S. consumers spend $2 million a year on posies.[42] However, since we do not normally eat flowers (more on edible flowers later), most people are not as concerned about the growing conditions or chemicals of flowers as they are with their food. In addition, most flowers don't come with a label other than a variety name, so the details of their origin and cultivation methods remain a mystery. Consumer expectations of perfect, long-lasting flowers mean that they come laden with chemicals to kill insects, fungi, etc. Demand for out-of-season flowers, like roses in winter, has shifted

---

42   Mark, Jason. "Unhealthy Flowers – why buying organic should not end with your food." *AlterNet,* February 13, 2007.

the modern flower industry to Central and South America where flowers can be grown year-round.

Flowers, like our foods, have changed greatly in our lifetimes. Tinkering with natural systems sometimes brings improvements, but modern science can also get carried away and take those enhancements to an undesirable level. Flower aficionado Amy Stewart writes in her book *Flower Confidential*, "There's no doubt that flowers underwent a complete makeover in the twentieth century. ...Thanks to those advances, there are some fantastic flowers on the market, all year long, for a remarkably cheap price. But modern flowers have lost something, too. They're tamer, better behaved, less fickle, and less seasonal. Many have lost their scent, and I wondered if they were also losing their identity, their power or their passion."[43] As consumers, we need to think about what qualities we really want in our bouquets and be careful that our desires don't unwittingly encourage scientists to remove more of the characteristics that flowers ought to have.

FOREIGN FLOWERS

While California is the largest domestic floral supplier in the United States, three-fourths of our nation's cut flowers are imported. Most come from massive greenhouses in Latin America but the United States also imports flowers from Holland, Thailand, and Kenya. Flowers from equatorial regions provide us with colorful centerpieces at Christmas, express our love on Valentine's Day, and allow us to shower our mothers with blooms on Mother's Day—all times when the North American climate limits the availability of abundant fresh-cut flowers. Yet what are the hidden costs?

> "*Flowers are created in laboratories, bred in test tubes, grown in factories, harvested by machines, packed into boxes, sold at auctions, and then flown across oceans and continents.*"
> — *Stewart*

Raising flowers this way requires heavy-duty pesticides that are both a hazard to the environment and a threat to worker safety. According to a 2007 AlterNet article, a survey of workers on Colombian flower plantations documented exposure to 127 different pesticides,

---

43   Stewart, Amy. *Flower Confidential: The Good, the Bad and the Beautiful.* (Algonquin Books: 2008) 8.

including three classified as extremely toxic. South American greenhouses frequently use chemicals that have been restricted or banned in the United States and Europe. To make matters worse, many of the workers are not provided with proper protective gear and suffer from impaired vision, respiratory and neurological problems as a result. Women in this industry also have high rates of stillbirths and babies born with congenital malformations.[44] U.S. florists also report irritation and dermatitis from contact with chemical-laden flowers.

Fortunately, it is possible to find reputable growers who care about worker safety. Increasing demand for organic flowers and the introduction of Veriflora certification (which specifies unacceptable chemicals and sets responsible labor and environmental standards) are motivating more growers to change. So if you are going to purchase commercial flowers, these labels are ways to ensure that your purchase has minimal ecological impact. However, even when grown under environmentally sound conditions, all cut flowers are heavy oil drinkers requiring a quick flight in the belly of a plane to reach Miami or New York and then a refrigerated road trip to their final destination.

The issue of avoiding floral purchases from abroad is a complex one, since the floral industry does provide much-needed jobs in poorer countries. Nevertheless, one still wonders if decreased demand for flower and food exports would stimulate a local economy to flourish in these places, producing goods desperately needed within those communities.

GO NATURAL

So if a genetically modified carnation or rose dipped in fungicide doesn't express your true feelings for your loved one, what are your options? Like vegetables, flowers are seasonal. Tulips and daffodils in spring, zinnias, snapdragons, and sunflowers for summer, and mums with pumpkins in fall are seasonal possibilities. Evergreen arrangements can even solve the Christmas dilemma. Admittedly, Valentine's Day does present a larger hurdle if you are seeking truly local blossoms that are fresh and not dried, but there are alternatives,

---

44   Mark, Jason. "Unhealthy Flowers – why buying organic should not end with your food." *AlterNet*, February 13, 2007.

like choosing a potted plant from a local greenhouse. If the chemical residue on bouquets you intend to bury your nose in is a concern, choosing flowers from a local grower gives you better opportunity to investigate growing practices.

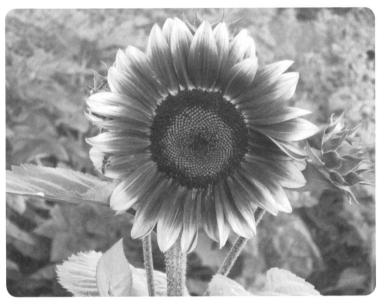

Local flowers are a graceful addition to a locally grown meal. Tucking a bouquet into your farmers' market basket provides food for both body and soul.

One flower farm in our area offers a more sustainable option to long-distance flowers. The Miller family grows over an acre of annuals and perennials on their family farm. They start seedlings in their greenhouse, which is heated by burning scrap wood from their woodworking shop. Tilling is done with their team of Percheron horses and an old-fashioned icehouse serves as a flower cooler. Their large family provides the labor for planting, weeding, and picking. An older daughter makes many of the bouquets, using over fifty varieties of cut flowers. Currently the majority of the Millers' sales are to a wholesaler, but they would like to expand their farm stand and sell directly to florists. The Millers were inspired by Lynn Byczynski's books and articles on raising flowers (see resources). Small-scale flower farms are beginning to bloom in many other areas thanks to Lynn's influence.

Another obstacle to overcome in choosing local flowers is using over fifty varieties of cut flowers including Bells of Ireland, snapdragons and celosia. We can thank Martha Stewart for helping to change this mindset by making forget-me-nots in a teacup and a handful of brilliant zinnias look fashionable. "Common" flowers, lovingly picked and uniquely arranged, can convey greater affection than their tropical cousins with longer vase lives. Some see the necessity of changing the table bouquet more often as an opportunity to experience even more beauty.

I am thankful to have a market-gardening friend with a knack for flower arranging. I loved all the delightful arrangements she brought to church and especially the different varieties of sunflowers that grow in her garden. She could take the ordinary and arrange them into something extraordinary. When our 25th anniversary rolled around and my in-laws' 60th anniversary right behind in late summer, I didn't even consider store-bought flowers. I highly value our friendship and wanted to keep my dollars in the local market, rather than giving them to some chain store. The farm-fresh arrangements I bought were gorgeous, and a great value besides.

-Judy K. is a secretary who loves flowers. She surrounds her home with colorful bedding plants, but their wooded lot only allows one sunny corner for a single raised bed where she raises a small assortment of veggies.

With the availability of authentic-looking plastic and silk floral decorations, why bother with live flowers that shed pollen, wilt, and need to be replaced? Choosing live decorations helps reduce one's environmental footprint and supports a local farmer. Living pussy willow and forsythia branches help usher in spring in a way that silk alternatives cannot fully mimic, and a bouquet of fragrant fresh flowers during summer gives more aromatic pleasure than a pitcher of plastic posies. Many fall squashes are quite decorative and can later be turned into squash soup or pumpkin bread, while harvest decorations of seeds, sunflowers, and corn shocks are both beautiful and useful for feeding the birds. At the end of their life, these natural decorations will enrich your compost pile rather than taking up space in the landfill.

My uncle Clarence, a great gardener, said he grows food for the body and flowers for the soul. The satisfaction of flower gardening, like any gardening, comes from working together with my Creator and with my family. It brings together generations: my mom, my daughters, daughter-in-law, and granddaughter. There are few things as satisfying as planting tulip bulbs, or cutting zinnias and sunflowers with a granddaughter, who at five can put together beautiful arrangements. Then there is the satisfaction of sharing your flowers with shut-ins and those recovering from illness or as birthday or thank-you gifts. One friend who was recovering from surgery last summer said she really liked my homegrown bouquet because it didn't seem "funeral-y." I use recycled glass jars with a ribbon, or tin cans with tissue paper tied around them as containers—no one has to bother returning the vase.

There is probably a place for artificial or silk flowers, but we don't use them in our home. You can begin in March by forcing forsythia and cutting pussy willows, followed by daffodils and tulips, bleeding hearts, crabapple blossoms, lilacs, iris, and lily-of-the-valley. Then it's summer, and you can have larger and brighter arrangements of annuals such as zinnias, cosmos, sunflowers, etc. I use Queen Anne's lace a lot. In fall, you can add goldenrod, "bluetops," and mums. To me, the greenery in a fresh arrangement is almost as important as the blossoms and I use Sweet Cicely, cosmos greens, daylily leaves, ivy, and pine branches.

With a little effort, you can have something fresh in your home through November. Then gather bittersweet, seedpods, fresh greens, and pinecones to take you through the winter. And you haven't purchased any imports or used any chemicals or fuel.

-Leanna D. is a grandmother who appreciates her natural surroundings. In addition to her extensive perennial beds, her family recently added 4000 trees to their property.

FINDING LOCAL FLOWERS

An excellent source for local flowers is the farmers' market, where many vendors have a few vases tucked among their wares and you will often find a "Flower Lady" specializing in flowers. Master gardener Dee B. and her daughter, Joanna, are a floral team who run a flower booth at a Saturday morning farmers' market in a city of about 40,000. Buckets of zinnias, snapdragons, celosia, statice, and sunflowers (their most popular seller) fill their car trunk and tables along with some unusual varieties like love-lies-bleeding and cockscomb. Joanna, a schoolteacher on summer vacation, handpicks stems to create a custom bouquet for each customer. Dee admits that one challenge of using the farmers' market as an outlet for their bouquets is the risk of a stormy Friday, which makes for ragged flowers, or a rainy Saturday, which can mean sluggish sales. Dee says, "We sell bouquets at the market because of our love of gardening, and flowers are a good outlet for sharing our blessings with others. We keep our prices reasonable so that we can spread our joy to many people and, in a sense, we are sharing a part of our farmland with others."

Finding locally grown flowers may require a little detective work. You might find a seasonal florist or home-based grower or inquire at a florist shop about the source of their flowers, suggesting that they offer local options in season. Several family-owned mail order companies carry natural decorations such as birdseed ornaments, dried arrangements, and holiday greenery decorations.

LOCAL FLOWERS FOR SPECIAL OCCASIONS

When their eldest daughter announced her engagement and wanted an outdoor wedding decorated with bright, colorful garden flowers, the Stoltzfus family started planting zinnias, sunflowers, cosmos, and dahlias to bloom in August. The day before the wedding, they gathered buckets of flowers from their own garden and from the gardens of grandmothers, neighbors, and even a few willing strangers along with some wildflowers. A florist friend transformed the orange, red, and yellow array into corsages, bridal bouquets, table arrangements in eclectic jars, and other cheerful decorations. "Growing your own wedding flowers is not for everyone," said the bride's mom. "Our dahlias bloomed two weeks late and an aunt had to go pick more wildflowers that morning to make sure everything was filled. But it worked for us because the bride was very flexible and many guests commented on how the wedding truly reflected the style of the bride (who walked down the aisle barefoot) and groom."

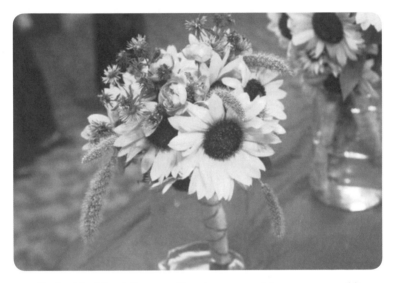

Fresh-picked local flowers add uniqueness and beauty to a wedding without the environmental cost of their long-distance relatives. The bride who carried this bouquet planned her wedding date around the availability of her favorite flowers. She grew some of them in her own garden and handed out seed packets to friends and relatives to add to the celebration.

I (Karen) love growing flowers in my market garden for their beauty and ability to attract beneficial insects, and allow my children to pick abundant bouquets for our home. When I am making bouquets to sell, I most enjoy arranging those for which I know the destination—a birthday gift for a mother, congratulations for a spouse's first publication, or a special anniversary.

It's also exciting to help grow flowers for wedding celebrations. I planted blue sweet peas this spring for a cousin's June wedding. An August bride-to-be requested an assortment of deep plum, orange, and white flowers, which involved scouring my seed catalogs for just the right shade. When we will be visiting someone with a birthday, our children instinctively go gather a colorful bouquet to give.

Flowers are such a natural and beautiful way to celebrate special events.

Our family attended calling hours one August for the elderly mother of a friend. I couldn't help noticing that the sympathy flowers covering the wall, though quite beautiful, were all sourced from thousands of miles away even though it was peak flower season in Ohio. I wondered if thoughtful arrangements of zinnias, snapdragons, and cosmos would have been a more appropriate tribute to this lady who was most certainly a gardener in her younger years.

At another summer funeral, the Gerber family contributed handpicked flowers to help honor their grandmother. The family collected flowers from neighbors, family, and fields, and included antique varieties from their grandmother's own flowerbed. The children and grandchildren gathered to help arrange a pastel casket spray made of phlox, Echinacea, snapdragons, hosta, Queen Anne's lace, etc. under the guidance of a granddaughter with some floral background. Family members said that working together on this project was helpful in the healing process, and guests noticed the special homemade touch in the arrangement.

GROWING YOUR OWN

Putting local flowers on your table can be as simple as plucking a few stems from your flowerbed, garden, or even the ditch. Adding a few short rows to your garden will supply you with plenty of blooms all summer long. Zinnias, tall snapdragons, sunflowers, and bachelor's buttons are good choices for ease of growing and longer vase life. A bed of perennial flowers will also yield cut flowers with the added bonus of not having to replant each year. Some good perennials for cutting include Echinacea, yarrow, ornamental grasses, and black-eyed Susans. Vases can simply be recycled glass jars or you can be creative and use antique bottles, teakettles, and pitchers. Don't forget to let children add their unique style to arranging flowers.

EDIBLE FLOWERS

Fresh flowers are not only for the vase—some are delightful additions to the dinner plate. Edible flowers are a prominent curiosity in high-end food establishments but can also dress up the family table. They can make a salad instantly glamorous, bring elegance to a wedding cake, or serve as a spicy addition to a vegetable dish. Easy-to-grow edible flowers include nasturtiums, calendula, Johnny jump-ups, chive blossoms, borage, and pea blossoms. Because of their fragile nature, a local source is about the only economical option for obtaining fresh-looking edible flowers and you want to be sure they are organically grown and properly identified. Rhoda G. says, "Receiving a handful of edible flowers in our weekly salad bag from the farm is a real treat. Some add flavor, others add beauty and make a simple salad into something extraordinary. The kids will even try them and when we have guests, they are amazed that you could actually eat flowers."

CONCLUSION

If you have made the choice to seek out local foods, flowers are a natural extension of that choice since they are often produced alongside food, under similar conditions. The beauty of seasonal flowers grown close to home goes well beyond appearances when you consider the larger issues behind your bouquet.

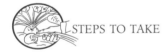STEPS TO TAKE

1. Look for local flowers at a farmers' market or find a flower-growing friend and enjoy the beauty, scent, and uniqueness of the flowers.

2. Add a row of cutting flowers to your garden or flowerbed for fresh bouquets from your backyard.

3. Ask your florist about the sources of flowers in their shop. When you do need to purchase there, look for organic options and keep bouquets seasonal (avoid tulips in October).

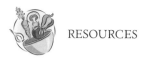

RESOURCES

1. *Flower Confidential* by Amy Stewart
2. *The Flower Gardener's Bible* by Lewis and Nancy Hill
3. *The Flower Farmer* by Lynn Byczynski
4. *Edible Flowers from Garden to Palate* by Cathy Wilkinson Barash

HOW TO START AN EASY CUTTING GARDEN

A 4' x 8' raised bed or area in your garden will supply a profusion of cut flowers for your home and bouquets to share. Prepare and enrich the soil with compost as you would for vegetables. Below is a simple planting guide using easy-to-find, direct-seeded annual varieties. You may choose to substitute purchased plants from a greenhouse such as snapdragons, salvia, or celosia.

BACK ROW: Branching sunflowers ..... Cosmos (for both foliage and flowers)

MIDDLE ROW: Zinnias (Benary's Giant is an excellent variety)

FRONT ROW: Nasturtiums (an edible flower) ..... Love-in-a-Mist (seedpods are beautiful also)

Flowers are best cut in the morning just after the dew has dried, or in the evening. Use a clean, sharp scissors or clippers to cut stems and place in clean warm water for an hour or more to condition them. Strip bottom leaves and recut stems at an angle as you arrange them in a vase with a few drops of bleach in the water to inhibit bacterial growth. Change the water every other day to lengthen the vase life of your flowers.

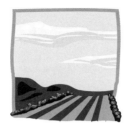

Chapter 12

Visions for the Future

A hundred years after we are gone and forgotten, those who never heard
of us will be living with the results of our actions.
-Oliver Wendell Holmes

THE FUTURE IS BRIGHT

The time is ripe for both farmers and consumers to transform our country. The local foods movement is being driven by some of the most unlikely folks—inner-city children growing gardens and chefs demanding the best ingredients; college students working for a better world and moms desiring healthy families; older folks remembering the way things "used to taste" and farmers seeking to earn an income doing what they passionately love. This diverse group is connected by the commonality of good food.

We believe that the future of the local foods movement is bright. Many factors are driving this movement, from fluctuating gas prices and food shortages to newly recognized health benefits and a longing for a sense of community. "From my experience, the only consumer group growing faster than 'organics' are the 'locavores' (people choosing a local conventional product over the organic product coming from far away)," reports Phil Nabors, owner of the Mustard Seed Market in northeastern Ohio.

The number of farmers' markets is steadily increasing each year. Many people are reconnecting with the people who grow their food, even if only in small ways, and others are returning to the land to grow their own. There are more options available in the United States than ever before. Consumer demand for cleaner foods will go a long way in redirecting industrial agriculture standards toward a safer food supply for everyone.

It is our dream to help develop a new type of food culture, in our neighborhood and elsewhere—a culture where not everyone has to grow their own dinner, but where they still feel a connection with the land and with the farmers who do grow that dinner; a local foodshed that encourages a sense of community, with neighbors feeding neighbors.

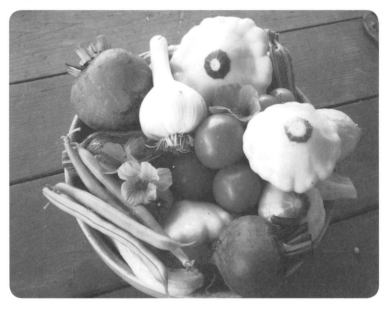

Our vision for the future of local foods includes a bountiful harvest that blesses both farmers and consumers, reaches all economic levels and deepens our sense of community.

I would love to see more people eating seasonally and to have a local CSA where we could have lots of people get involved and "own" their food sources. I want my children to know how and where the things on our table come from so they can in turn share with those they come into contact with. I also really am excited about what is currently happening and want to make more people aware of it.

-*Jennifer S.*

TAKING OWNERSHIP

A first step toward accomplishing this vision is for everyone to take more ownership in their food choices. For some, this will mean growing some of their own, and for others, knowing more intimately where their meat, milk, grains, and veggies are coming from. The assumption that government regulations and grocery store systems will always keep us healthy and well fed needs to be challenged. Local food systems offer a true freedom that returns us to the roots of our country, so rich in agricultural resources. They are something that everyone can take part in; young or old, urban or rural, regardless of race, politics, or religion.

Food can bring us together in many positive ways. An Amish farmer shared with us, "I'm not very optimistic about the food system in America, but I'm very optimistic about the people that are opting out of the industrial food system. These people know what they are doing and why they're doing it."

> We own a natural foods store that has over 30,000 customers and sells many truckloads of produce each week, but we still grow a garden. Our family lives in the city and grows veggies and fruit. We even have a greenhouse. It's important for us to participate in growing our food and we want our children to know that their food comes from the earth.
>
> -Phil N., *owner of Mustard Seed Market*

IN THE CITY

We dream of cities that are not concrete jungles but green, productive places jam-packed with trees, gardens, and even small livestock such as chickens, honeybees, and rabbits. And indeed, exciting things are happening in cities across the country. Urban farmers are discovering that small, intensive farming plots can be quite profitable, since minimal transport is necessary and freshness is optimized (see www.spinfarming.com). Schools are even getting in on the act with programs like The Edible Schoolyard—planting gardens and letting the children help to grow their own lunches.

My vision is that city folk would have the desire and resources to plant a small garden in their backyard. That whole foods could be available to them year-round...as organic as possible! That more farmers could have a market for and make a good profit from their organic foods. People that run city shops could also make a living knowing that their customers are happy and can afford to pay for the quality produce.

-*Ramona N.*

FOR SUBURBIA

Despite all the criticism it receives, suburbia actually has a lot of potential. Suburbanites just need to "stop mowing and start growing!" If large suburban lawns were converted to food production, they would become useful as well as beautiful. Larger yards could easily support some small livestock—chickens, goats, sheep, or bees—in addition to fruit trees, berries, and gardens. A number of books from the 1970s homesteading movement list ways to grow food in one's backyard. One of these, *The Have More Plan,* recently went back into print and contains plans for a 1-acre, 2-acre, or 5-acre homestead. The USDA has written another helpful guide, entitled *Living on an Acre.*

Eventually it would be wonderful if many people went back to growing at least a few things on their own property—even people who live in town. More lawns could be turned into small gardens. People could feel it was acceptable to have food in place of a lawn or to have a couple of fruit trees or grapevines. People in cities and small towns can also do container gardening and participate in community gardens where there are small plots that are free or available for a small rental fee. I'd hope that in the future everyone could identify where most of their food was grown and that the bulk of it would have come from the state they live in and even from people they know in their own communities.

For those who are interested in learning, there might be a resurgence of classes in food preparation and food preservation for fun, economy, and nutrition. This could be especially beneficial to people on fixed incomes and low-income families who currently subsist on highly processed food. Transportation services and a local food voucher could allow low-income people in cities to enjoy the bounty of nearby rural areas.

-Joanne L.

If you have a yard, why not make your landscaping edible rather than purely ornamental? Choose a fruit or nut tree, a berry bush, or even edible flowers instead of conventional alternatives for a lawn that is both beautiful and productive. Most suburbanites—homeowners' association rules aside—could easily raise a significant portion of their own food in their own backyard. Gardening and tending animals can be a great way to spend quality family time together and to teach children useful skills.

I'd like to see more heritage varieties of fruits and vegetables; more heritage breeds; and more small enterprises such as cheese makers, goat farms, and fruit and nut farms. I'd also like to see more restaurants with a commitment to local and seasonal offerings collaborating with small area producers and artisans; large areas in supermarkets devoted to and featuring locally grown products; education and festivals celebrating the rich diversity of locally grown and produced foods and delicacies; and financial subsidies for expansion and growth.

-Monique T.

FOR THE COUNTRYSIDE

Farmers, many of whom have struggled mightily just to stay in business and who have been unfairly stigmatized for decades, stand to benefit greatly from the local foods movement. We hope that as more people begin to spend their food dollars locally, farming won't need to be just a "hobby" supported by outside employment but will again become a respected and profitable occupation.

We consider ourselves fortunate to live in Amish country, where through a combination of theology and geography, farms have tended to remain small and diverse. A patchwork of different crops, grazing animals, and human habitations create a varied and interesting landscape, in sharp contrast to the huge monocultures of corn and beans grown in other parts of the Midwest. Small towns in this area continue to thrive, also in contrast to much of the Midwest, where the population has plummeted as farmland has been consolidated into the hands of fewer and fewer landowners. Amish country stands as a reminder of how things used to be, when people supported their local economies by necessity, and how things could be again in the rest of rural America. But these visions are not limited to areas already thriving with small-scale agriculture. It's not too late to invigorate your neighborhood with a new zeal for good food. Perhaps you can encourage people affected by unemployment to consider agriculture or help start a community garden, buying group, or even a farmers' market in your area.

> I think there's a place for farmers to be full-time farmers and grow food for American families again, and I would like to see our culture support that, but I think it's going to be a long time in the making. It starts with people that are willing to do it on the side to get it going and create a market where they can sell enough and make enough money to survive. And the restaurants have to be willing to see the value in it and pay because you can buy an apple through the conventional food system that's much cheaper—but it won't be the same quality.
>
> -*Mike M.*

GOING BEYOND

We have presented some of our ideas here, but we hope that you will come up with your own new and creative solutions to any barriers you may face in your region in finding and eating local foods. A recent *New York Times* article listed a variety of creative options for the "lazy locavore," such as the FruitGuys, a company in San Francisco and Philadelphia that delivers boxes of local and sustainable fruit to the office, and Three Stone Hearth in Berkeley, a community-supported kitchen where customers can gather to cook local foods together. Some wealthy homeowners are even hiring gardeners to plant, tend, and harvest gardens in their own backyards so they can have the benefits of a garden without the work. Customers in some areas can now have canned goods or even fully cooked meals delivered to their homes. Others are purchasing shares in cows (for beef or milk) and pigs—a practice known as "cow pooling" or "herdshares."[45]

> My vision for the future is that all basic foods in our diet could be obtained locally, and that there would be resources available to make them easier to find. While it would be costly and I can't presently afford it, I would love in the future to have all the food that I purchase be produced within a 5-15-mile radius. (That would of course require further changes in our family's diet to eliminate all processed foods, and we're gradually working on that.) I'm not sure how things like stevia powder, baking powder/soda, yeast, and other such foods could be handled locally. I would love to see regulatory controls loosened to make things like raw milk and unpasteurized cider legally available.
>
> *-Jolene M.*

CONCLUSION

If the local food concept is new to you, we hope this book has inspired you to at least try a few "local choices." Perhaps that means making a single purchase. If you are ready to take a bigger bite, you can commit to making one meal a week centered on local foods. If you're ready to chew off even more, you might want to set a goal of spending a certain percentage of your grocery budget on foods grown close to home, or choosing a percentage of food that you want to attempt growing on your own.

We heartily agree with the words of one of our contributors: "I hope more people catch on to the fun and satisfaction of local eating

---

45   Severson, Kim. "A Locally Grown Diet with Fuss but No Muss," *New York Times*, July 22, 2008. www.nytimes.com/2008/07/22/dining/22local.html?scp=1&sq=lazy%20 locavores&st=cse

and gardening so that our food system can be healthier and more just for all who live and eat in it." *Bon appétit!*

TEN WAYS TO SPREAD THE WORD

1. Invite a friend to visit the farmers' market with you. In the process of writing this book, the authors took several fun "field trips" to area farmers' markets. We particularly enjoyed visiting a winter market in Cleveland one chilly Saturday—it was refreshing to smell the aroma of baked goods, and a pleasant surprise to see just how much food is still available in mid-winter—even in Cleveland. Vendors offered honey, apples, pea shoots, eggs, popcorn, canned items, and much more.

2. Get together with friends to make a giant batch of spaghetti sauce, can peaches, make strawberry jam or applesauce, etc. Many hands make light work, as my grandmother used to say.

3. Take a local dish to your next potluck meal, add local foods to your next party menu—and be sure to let your guests know where they came from. Or host a local foods party. One friend of ours hosted several seasonal brunches and asked each guest to bring a seasonal dish. Many people brought friends, so new friendships and connections were made.

4. Suggest that your book group read and discuss a book on local foods, or invite a local farmer to speak to your civic group or social club. Ask them to bring samples! Or consider offering to teach a class on eating local at your church, library, or community college.

5. Connect with other local foods aficionados in your area. Gather a Slow Food or Weston Price group, plan a cooking event or simply share iced tea at the farmer's market.

6. If you're a gardener, start a garden swap group. Karen organized a group one summer that met periodically during the harvest season to share "extras" with the others. The contributions were divvied up and each participant went home with a share of the bounty. It was a good occasion to

socialize and share gardening tips as well.

7. Next time you take someone special out for a meal, try a restaurant featuring local, seasonal foods.

8. Home-canned or dehydrated foods such as jams, salsa, sun-dried tomatoes, dried fruit, pickles, or chutney make lovely (and delicious) gifts. Use a pretty jar, tie with ribbon or raffia, and print some labels to create one-of-a-kind gifts from your kitchen this year.

9. Encourage a farmer—whether it be someone on a half-acre lot in town, a five-acre farmette, or 200 acres. As more people start eating local, we'll need more farmers to supply the demand.

10. Come visit and link to our blog at http://localchoices. wordpress.com. Last but certainly not least—share this book with family members or give one as a gift!

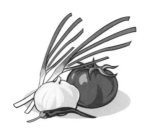

Appendix A: Recipes

Rhubarb Crunch

Lisa Amstutz

Topping:

1 C. flour
1 C. brown sugar
1 tsp. cinnamon

¾ C. uncooked oatmeal
½ C. butter, melted

Fruit:

4 C. rhubarb, diced
1 C. water
1 tsp. vanilla

1 C. white sugar
2 T. cornstarch

Mix topping together and put half of it into an 8 x 8" baking pan. Press it firmly on the bottom of the pan. Save the remaining topping.

Place rhubarb over crumbs in pan. Cook sugar, cornstarch, water, and vanilla until thick and clear. Stir constantly. Pour over rhubarb; top with remaining crumbs. Bake at 350° for one hour. Serve hot or cold with whipped cream or milk. Yield: 6 servings.

SWEDISH PANCAKE

AMY HEADINGS

Pan Size	Butter	Eggs	Milk	Flour
2-3 qt.	¼ C.	3	¾ C.	¾ C.
3-4 qt.	⅓ C.	4	1 C.	1 C.
4-4½ qt.	½ C.	5	1¼ C.	1¼ C.
4½-5 qt.	½ C.	6	1½ C.	1½ C.

Select the amount of ingredients and the size of your baking pan according to chart. The bigger and shallower the pan, the better. Figure one serving for each egg used. Melt butter in the baking pan in a 425° F. oven (400° for a glass pan). Put eggs into blender on high speed for one minute. Pour in milk while whirling, then add flour and blend for 30 seconds. Add ½ tsp. salt and blend 10 more seconds. Pour mix into pan and bake 25 minutes until it's puffed up and golden brown. Serve with maple syrup or confectioners' sugar, or if you want to be truly authentic, with Hollandaise sauce.

PITA PIZZA

Pita pizzas (or bread pizzas) are a fun and easy alternative to the processed pizza rolls or pockets sold in the grocery store. Simply start with a small pita or slice of bread for each person. Top with pizza sauce, cheese, and whatever other toppings you enjoy. Children may be more amenable to adding seasonal vegetables if you let them create faces or other designs with them.

SHISH KEBABS

Marinate the meat of your choice overnight for best flavor and tenderness. String chunks of meat (chicken, seafood, beef roast, or stew meat, etc.) on a bamboo or metal skewer, interspersed with a variety of vegetables—mushrooms, onions, green peppers, zucchini, summer squash, cherry tomatoes, carrots, and pineapple chunks are some of our favorites. Carrots need to be partially cooked ahead of time so they will slide easily onto the skewer. Grill until meat is done.

Flank Steak Marinade

½ C. soy sauce	½ C. vegetable oil
1 T. molasses	1 tsp. ginger
1 tsp. dry mustard	2-3 garlic cloves, minced

Marinate 3-6 hours in a self-sealing one-gallon bag. Shake every hour.

Mint Tea

Bring to a boil: 4 C. water, 2 C. sugar. Remove from heat. Wash 2 C. mint leaves and add to hot water. Allow to steep for several hours. Strain out mint leaves and add enough water and ice to make one gallon of tea. Other sweeteners may be substituted for sugar if desired.

Potato Wedges

Wash potatoes. Slice lengthwise into wedges (6 or 8 per potato). Arrange potatoes cut side up on a cookie sheet and brush with melted butter. Sprinkle with Parmesan or herbs to taste. Bake at 350° for 45 minutes or until tops are starting to crisp and brown. Serve with ketchup. (Sweet potatoes make good wedged fries as well.)

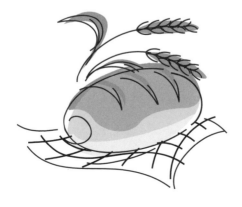

100% WHOLE WHEAT BREAD   LEORA GERBER

2 C. boiling water	2 eggs, beaten
½ C. powdered dry milk	7-8 C. whole-wheat flour
½ C. butter	(can be fresh ground)
1 tsp. salt	½ C. honey
2 T. yeast	

In a large bowl, pour boiling water over dry milk, butter, salt, and honey. Allow to cool to between 115-120° (use candy thermometer). Add dry yeast, beaten eggs, and 3 cups flour gradually and beat with electric mixer for about 5 minutes. Stir in another 2½ cups flour with wooden spoon. Turn dough onto floured board and knead, using flour sparingly until smooth and elastic, about 10 minutes. Cover dough ball with towel and let rest 20 minutes. Punch down by kneading a few strokes. Divide into 4 parts. Roll out with rolling pin in rectangle shape and roll up jellyroll fashion to shape loaves. Put in bread pans and let rise until double. Bake at 350° for 30-35 minutes. Makes 4 loaves.

BUTTER

Watching cream transform into butter is something everyone should experience at least once. It is a fun project to do with children, taking turns with the shaking.

Ingredients: 1 pint heavy cream or whipping cream (be careful not to use "ultra pasteurized")

Bring cream to room temperature. Pour into a quart canning jar with tight-fitting lid and shake vigorously until butter forms (15-20 minutes). You can also use a blender or food processor. Pour off buttermilk and save it for recipes like pancakes (see following recipe). Rinse the butter with cold water to expel additional buttermilk. Add salt to taste. For a more exotic flavor, you can mix in herbs like chopped rosemary with minced shallots or chives. The herbal butters are delicious on hot sweet corn, fresh bread, or crackers.

BUTTERMILK PANCAKES

MIX:

2 T. melted butter	2 eggs
2 T. sugar	1 tsp. baking powder
1 tsp. cinnamon	pinch of salt
1 C. whole wheat flour	1 C. rolled oats
(we use fresh ground)	
2 C. buttermilk	
Optional – 1 C. fresh or frozen berries	

Pour onto griddle and cook until golden brown. Delicious served with maple syrup.

SOFT HERBED CHEESE

Heat 1 gallon milk to 90°. Add 1 tablespoon of yogurt or a packet of direct-set mesophilic starter plus 3-4 drops liquid rennet (available from cheese supply houses) and stir gently. Cover and let set in warm area for 12 hours or until a solid curd forms. Pour into a cheesecloth bag and hang to drain for 6-12 hours. Whey can be used in recipes, fed to pets, or used as garden fertilizer. Add salt and herbs (rosemary/shallot, dill/chives, oregano/garlic, etc.) as desired. Shape into a cheese ball or log shape and garnish with herbs or edible flowers. Keeps 1-2 weeks in the refrigerator. Use this delicious spread on crackers or bread.

Lamb Curry   Gillian Berchowitz

This recipe is based on one from Van Wyk, Magdaleen, and Pat Barton. *Traditional South African Cooking*. Cape Town: Struik, 2007.

While there are plenty of recipes for grilled or broiled loin or rib chops and roasted racks of lamb, the shoulder and sirloin chops and steaks, ribs, or top round are best cut up into chunks (with or without the bone), fat removed, and cooked slowly for 60 to 90 minutes until the sauce is well melded and the meat is tender.

This traditional South African lamb curry was inspired by Malay recipes brought to Cape Town by prisoners and slaves of the Dutch East India Company. These sweeter mild curries are a treasured centerpiece of traditional South African cooking.

Combine in a small bowl:

½ tsp. ground cinnamon	1 tsp. ground coriander
¼ tsp. ground cumin	2 cloves garlic, crushed
2 T. curry powder	1½ T. cake flour
1 tsp. turmeric	

Prepare 3 lbs. lamb rib, shoulder, sirloin, or stewing cuts by trimming excess fat. Cut the shoulder chops into thirds or smaller pieces and cube the other meat into uniform chunks, with or without the bone. I like to keep the bones as they add flavor and one can gauge doneness by when the meat begins to fall off the bone.

2 T. sunflower oil
2 large onions, finely chopped
1 bay leaf
1 lb. medium tomatoes, skinned and chopped
6-8 dried peaches, apricots, finely chopped, or ½ cup raisins
2 T. fruit chutney—any bottled brand will do. South Africans
    look for Mrs. Ball's Chutneys, which is available in the U.S.
1 C. meat (beef) stock
1 tsp. white sugar
2 tsp. salt
freshly ground black pepper

Heat the oil in a large saucepan and sauté the onions for about 5 minutes, or until transparent. Add the bay leaf, cinnamon, coriander, cumin, garlic, curry powder, flour, and turmeric, and simmer for a few minutes, stirring constantly. Add the meat and brown it lightly, adding a little more oil if necessary. Add the remaining ingredients and mix well. Simmer over moderate heat for 1 to 1½ hours. Serve immediately with boiled rice and bowls of sliced banana, desiccated coconut, diced pineapple, and chutney. This curry also keeps very well in the refrigerator and can be made in advance for company or family dinners. It makes excellent leftovers. Serves 6.

Sausage Apple Casserole   Susan Mark Landis

1 lb. ground sausage, browned and drained
3-4 apples, sliced
⅓ C. all-purpose flour
½ C. brown sugar
¼ C. butter
½ lb. cheddar cheese, sliced
¼ C. plain yogurt

Combine flour, brown sugar, and butter and use a pastry blender to make crumbs.

Layer in a casserole in this order: ground sausage, sliced apples, crumbs, cheddar cheese, and dollops of yogurt. Bake at 350° for approximately 30 minutes, until bubbly and browned on top.

Serving suggestion: Served with fresh bread or baked potatoes and baked winter squash, this meal will warm a chilly winter evening.

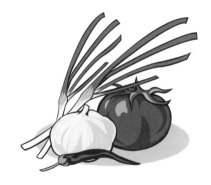

STIR-FRY BASICS   KAREN GEISER

When stir-fry is on the menu for supper, I get out a small package of meat to thaw in the morning. Vegetable combinations are often the result of a quick trip through the garden with a basket or using up a mixture of vegetables waiting in the refrigerator. Fresh herbs from my edible flowerbed give flavor. For a vegetarian meal, simply omit the meat.

> MEAT OPTIONS: ½ – 1# of: chicken breast or thigh, beef roast or sirloin, lamb or goat pieces
>
> VEGETABLE COMBO IDEAS:
>
> SPRING — snow peas, sweet onions, garlic scapes
>
> SUMMER — baby zucchini, colorful bell peppers, Swiss chard, lemon basil or French-cut green beans, cabbage, onions, thyme
>
> FALL — broccoli florets, leeks, kale

Cut meat into small pieces. If there is time, marinate meat in a vinaigrette or soy sauce mixture. Heat olive oil in a large skillet and cook meat until browned. Add chopped vegetables and salt to taste and stir-fry several minutes until crisp tender. Tender greens like kale, chard, and herbs should be added near the end and cooked until bright green.

If you want a sauce, mix 2 T. cornstarch into 1 cup broth, add to the skillet at the end, and cook until thickened.

Serve over rice or as a vegetable side dish.

GRILLED PATTY PANS   RACHEL GEISER

Gently wash Patty Pans and slice them (¼" thick) or cut into wedges. Toss them with olive oil and salt and pepper to taste. Preheat grill, then grill squash until crisp tender. Set aside to cool and prepare the following vinaigrette:

VINAIGRETTE DRESSING

Heat in a pan on the stove until the sugar is dissolved:

| ¾ C. cider vinegar | 6 T. sugar |

ADD:

| ¼ tsp. garlic powder | salt and pepper to taste |
| fresh herbs | |

Drizzle in 4 T. olive oil as you combine all ingredients.

Add your grilled squash, plus optional vegetables (onions, carrots, peppers) to the vinaigrette and use it as a side dish or on a bed of lettuce as a salad topper.

SLOW COOKER POTATOES WITH TOPPINGS   KAREN GEISER

Our favorite way to make baked potatoes is in the slow cooker. All we do is wash the potatoes (we like Buttes and Yukon Gold best) and fill the slow cooker. Three to four hours on high will produce beautiful and moist potatoes. We serve them with toppings like chili sauce (browned hamburger plus home-canned spaghetti sauce), steamed broccoli, and shredded cheese. Topped with chopped chives and our own sour cream they make a tasty and filling meal.

PASTA PRIMAVERA

KRIS SHANK ZEHR

1 sweet onion
1 zucchini (8")
1 stalk broccoli
1 tsp. dried basil or 1 T. fresh
olive oil

2-4 garlic cloves
1 yellow squash (8")
1 ripe tomato
8 oz. rotini

Cook pasta, drain, and set aside. Chop vegetables. Sauté onion, garlic, zucchini, and yellow squash in 2-4 T. olive oil. Add broccoli florets after 1-2 minutes. After five minutes, add tomatoes and basil. Stir into pasta. Serve with grated Parmesan, Asiago, Gruyère, or Fontanella cheese.

PEAR ZUCCHINI BREAD

ROXIE RAMSEYER

2 C. chopped, peeled pears
1 C. shredded zucchini
1 C. sugar
1 C. packed brown sugar
3 eggs, beaten
1 C. vegetable oil
1 T. vanilla

2 C. flour
1 C. rye or whole wheat flour
2 tsp. pumpkin pie spice
1 tsp. baking soda
½ tsp. baking powder
½ tsp. salt
½ C. chopped pecans

Combine the first seven ingredients. Combine flours, pie spice, soda, baking powder, and salt; stir into pear mixture until blended. Fold in nuts. Pour into two greased 8" x 4" x 2" loaf pans. Bake at 350° for 55-65 min. or until toothpick comes out clean. Cool in pans for 10 minutes; remove to a wire rack to cool completely. Yield: 2 loaves.

GARLIC PICKLES

LISA ZUERCHER

SYRUP:

2 C. cider vinegar
3 C. sugar

2 C. water

In quart jar, put slice of onion, clove of garlic, and a dill sprig. Slice cucumbers and pack in jar. Add $1/8$ tsp. alum and 1 tsp. salt per jar. Fill with syrup. Process 20 minutes in boiling water bath.

CREAMED SPINACH LISA AMSTUTZ

3 T. butter
¼ tsp. salt
1 C. milk
8 C. fresh spinach, chopped

2 T. flour
⅛ t. pepper
6 green onions, chopped

Wash spinach, chop, and put in saucepan. Cook over medium heat until spinach is wilted. Set aside. In a skillet, melt butter and sauté green onions until clear. Shake flour and milk together until flour is dissolved, and add slowly into the butter and onion mixture, stirring constantly until thickened. Add spinach, salt, and pepper to taste. Yield: 3-4 servings.

BURNT HONEY AND ORANGE VINAIGRETTE DEB GEISER

YIELD: 1 CUP

4 T. honey
2 tsp. orange zest
1½ T. vegetable oil
½ C. fresh orange juice

4 T. sherry wine vinegar
1 T. olive oil
salt and pepper to taste

Pour the honey into a non-stick skillet or saucepan. Cook on medium heat until it begins to foam up, and then reduce heat slightly and cook 4 to 5 minutes, swirling the pan occasionally, or the honey begins to caramelize and turn a light brown. Remove from heat and pour in the orange juice. Place over a low heat and let the honey dissolve. Stir in the orange zest and set aside to let the mixture cool (about 10 minutes). Whisk in vinegar, salt, pepper, and the oils until thickened and blended. Refrigerate until ready to use.

HOT PEPPER MUSTARD ROXIE RAMSEYER

36 banana peppers (or 8-9 C. semi-hot and 6-8 chilis
    or 3-4 cayenne peppers)
1 qt. yellow mustard
5 C. sugar

1 qt. white or cider vinegar
1 T. salt

Grind peppers finely. Add other ingredients. Bring to a boil, stirring occasionally. Make paste of 2 C. water and ½ C. flour. Stir in peppers until thick. Seal in hot jars. Makes approximately 12 pints.

BULGOGI

CORRIE YODER

1¼ lb. tender beef steak, sliced thinly
½ hard pear, chopped coarsely
4-5 garlic cloves, crushed
2" cube fresh ginger, peeled and chopped finely
4 T. soy sauce
5 mushrooms, sliced

cooked rice or noodles

1 medium-sized onion, thinly sliced
3 scallions, thinly sliced
1 medium-sized carrot, sliced
2 T. sesame oil
1 T. sesame seeds, toasted
2½ T. granulated sugar

Slice beef across grain and set aside in large bowl. Blend pear, garlic, ginger, and soy sauce in blender. Add to meat. Add the remaining ingredients, mix, cover, and refrigerate 1-24 hours (the longer the better).

Heat a large frying pan with a little oil. Pick the pieces of marinated meat out of the bowl and place one layer of them in the frying pan. Turn slices over as soon as they brown. Remove slices and set them aside as soon as you consider them done. Do not overcook. Continue cooking layers of the beef until all of the meat is done. Place the veggies and the rest of the sauce in the pan to cook briefly. Add the meat again and cook only long enough to reheat the meat. Serve over rice or noodles.

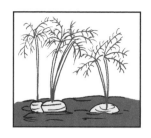

Appendix B: A Quick Guide to Vegetable and Fruit Storage and Preservation

Vegetable Name	Fresh Storage	Long-term Storage
Asparagus	*Ends in water in fridge (2-3 days)*	F,C
Beets	*Plastic bag in fridge (several weeks)*	R,L,C
Broccoli, Cauliflower	*Plastic bag in fridge (2 weeks)*	F
Cabbage	*Plastic bag in fridge (2 weeks)*	R,L,C
Carrots, Radishes, Turnips	*Plastic bag in fridge (several weeks)*	R
Corn	*Refrigerate in husks (1-2 days)*	F, L, C, D
Cucumbers	*Plastic bag in fridge (1 week)*	C, L
Eggplant	*Countertop (several days)*	F
Green Beans	*Plastic bag in fridge (several days)*	F, L, C, D
Lettuce	*Plastic bag in fridge (1 week)*	---------
Kale, Spinach, Chard, Collards	*Plastic bag in fridge (1 week)*	F
Okra	*Plastic bag in fridge (2-3 days)*	F,D
Onions, Garlic	*Cool, place in mesh bag (several month)*	D
Peas	*Plastic bag in fridge (several days)*	F, C
Peppers	*Plastic bag in fridge (1 week)*	F, C, D
Potatoes	*Cool, dark place (several weeks)*	R
Sweet Potatoes	*Cool, dark place, wrap in newspaper (several weeks)*	R
Summer Squash	*Plastic bag in fridge (1 week)*	F, C
Tomatoes	*Countertop (several days)*	F, C, D
Winter Squash	*Cool, dry place (several weeks-months)*	---------

FRUIT NAME	FRESH STORAGE	LONG-TERM STORAGE
Apples	*Plastic bag in fridge (several weeks)*	R, C, F, D
Blueberries	*Covered in fridge (1 week)*	C, F, D
Cherries	*Covered in fridge (2 days)*	C, F, D
Citrus	*Mesh bag in fridge (2 weeks)*	---------
Grapes	*Plastic bag in fridge (1 week)*	C, F, D
Melons	*Room temperature till fully ripe, then refrigerate (1 week)*	D
Peaches	*Cool place (1 week)*	C, F, D
Pears	*Room temp. until ripe, then fridge*	C, F, D
Plums	*Plastic bag in fridge (1 week)*	C, F, D
Raspberries/Blackberries	*Covered in fridge (2 days)*	C, F, D
Strawberries	*Covered in fridge (2 days)*	F, D

Key:
F = Freeze, C = Can, R = Root cellar,
L = Lacto-ferment, D = Dehydrate

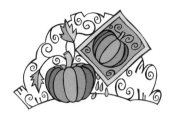

Appendix C: What's in Season?

This table is a general guide to when you may find items at the farmers' market. Availability will vary by region.

	SPRING	**SUMMER**	**AUTUMN**	**WINTER**
Apples		X	X	X
Arugula	X	X	X	
Asparagus	X			
Basil	X	X		
Beets		X	X	X
Berries		X		
Broccoli		X	X	
Brussels Sprouts			X	
Cabbage		X	X	X
Carrots		X	X	X
Cauliflower			X	
Celery		X	X	
Cherries		X		
Citrus				X
Collards			X	
Corn		X	X	
Cranberries			X	
Cucumbers		X		

	SPRING	SUMMER	AUTUMN	WINTER
Edamame		X		
Eggplant		X		
Garlic		X	X	X
Grapes			X	
Green Beans		X	X	
Honey	X	X	X	X
Leeks	X	X	X	
Lettuce	X		X	
Kale	X		X	X
Kohlrabi		X	X	
Melons		X	X	
Maple Syrup	X	X	X	X
Mint	X	X	X	
Okra		X		
Onions	X	X	X	X
Parsnips			X	X
Peaches		X		
Pears		X	X	
Peas	X		X	
Peppers		X	X	
Persimmons			X	
Plums		X		
Potatoes		X	X	X
Pumpkin			X	
Radishes	X		X	
Rhubarb	X			
Rutabagas			X	X
Spinach	X		X	
Strawberries	X			
Summer Squash		X		
Sweet Potatoes			X	X
Swiss Chard	X	X	X	
Tomatoes		X	X	
Turnips			X	X
Winter Squash			X	X
Wild Greens	X			

About the Authors

Karen Geiser, her husband Olin and five children are the sixth generation to live on a 78-acre diversified farm near Kidron, Ohio. They are in their eighth year of market gardening and grow salad greens, heirloom vegetables, herbs, and cut flowers. The Geisers also raise grass-fed beef, pastured poultry, goats, and free-range eggs.

The Geisers take seriously their task of caring for God's creation and have a passion for experimentation, education, and building community. When not digging blue potatoes, trying new kimchi recipes, or making cheese, Karen enjoys sharing her gardening knowledge through weekly demonstrations at Lehman's in Kidron, Ohio, and other speaking events. Karen holds a B.S. in Biology from Goshen College (IN), but says her most valuable education comes from digging in the dirt. She keeps a weekly garden journal on their farm website at www.karensgarden.net.

Lisa Amstutz is a freelance writer and mother of four. Ten years ago, she and her husband Michael bought an old farmhouse on six acres. Their Old MacDonald-style barnyard often slows traffic as drivers lean out to watch the turkeys or goats. They raise much of their own produce, meat, milk, and honey, and search out local sources for the rest whenever possible. Lisa also enjoys reading, scrapbooking, and spending time in nature.

Lisa has a B.S. in Biology from Goshen College (IN) and an M.S. in Environmental Science from the University of Virginia. Her articles and poetry have been published in a variety of magazines for children and adults. She writes regularly for Graphic Publications and is currently working on two nonfiction picture books to be published in 2011. Lisa blogs at http://ljamstutz.wordpress.com.